Allen's Fertil
Obstetrics in t

LIBRARY OF VETERINARY PRACTICE

EDITORS

J.B. SUTTON, JP, MRCVS

S.T. SWIFT, MA, VetMB, CertSAC

LIBRARY OF VETERINARY PRACTICE

Allen's Fertility and Obstetrics in the Horse

Second Edition

GARY C.W. ENGLAND
BVetMed, PhD, FRCVS, CertVA, DVR, DVReprod Diplomate ACT
Department of Farm Animal and Equine Medicine and Surgery
Royal Veterinary College, University of London
Hawkshead Lane, North Mymms
Hatfield, Herts

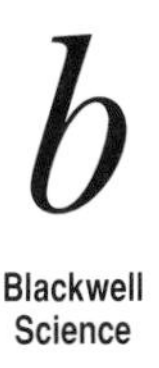

Blackwell
Science

Editorial Offices:
Osney Mead, Oxford OX2 0EL
25 John Street, London WC1N 2BL
23 Ainslie Place, Edinburgh EH3 6AJ
238 Main Street, Cambridge
Massachusetts 02142, USA
54 University Street, Carlton
Victoria 3053, Australia

Other Editorial Offices:
Arnette Blackwell SA
224, Boulevard Saint Germain
75007 Paris, France

Blackwell Wissenschafts-Verlag GmbH
Kurfürstendamm 57
10707 Berlin, Germany

Zehetnergasse 6
A-1140 Wien
Austria

First edition published 1988 as *Fertility and Obstetrics in the Horse* by W. Edward Allen
Reprinted 1989, 1991
Second edition published 1996

Set in 10 on 12 pt Souvenir
by DP Photosetting, Aylesbury, Bucks
Printed and bound in Great Britain at
the University Press, Cambridge

DISTRIBUTORS

Marston Book Services Ltd
PO Box 269
Abingdon
Oxon OX14 4YN
(*Orders:* Tel: 01235 465500
Fax: 01235 465555)

USA
Blackwell Science, Inc.
238 Main Street
Cambridge, MA 02142
(*Orders:* Tel: 800 215-1000
617 876-7000
Fax: 617 492-5263)

Canada
Copp Clark, Ltd
2775 Matheson Blvd East
Mississauga, Ontario
Canada, L4W 4P7
(*Orders:* Tel: 800 263-4374
905 238-6074)

Australia
Blackwell Science Pty Ltd
54 University Street
Carlton, Victoria 3053
(*Orders:* Tel: 03 9347 0300
Fax: 03 9347 5001)

A catalogue record for this title is available from the British Library

ISBN 0-632-04084-X

Library of Congress
Cataloging-in-Publication Data
England, Gary C.W.
Allen's fertility and obstetrics in the horse.—2nd ed./Gary C.W. England.
p. cm.—(Library of veterinary practice)
Rev. ed. of: Fertility and obstetrics in the horse/W. Edward Allen. 1988.
Includes bibliographical references and index.
ISBN 0-632-04084-X
1. Horses—Fertility. 2. Horses—Reproduction. 3. Veterinary obstetrics. 4. Veterinary gynecology. I. Allen, W. Edward. Fertility and obstetrics in the horse. II. Title. III. Series.
SF768.2.H67E54 1996
636.1'08982—dc20 96-24286
CIP

Contents

Preface

The author of the first edition of this book was my teacher, colleague and friend, the late Dr W. Edward Allen. Ed, as he wished to be known, wrote the book primarily for veterinary students, and veterinary surgeons who wanted to learn about equine stud practice. He used his great depth of knowledge and enthusiasm, based upon 20 years of experience, to produce a practical up-to-date text in which information was presented in a concise and readily accessible format. With Ed's death the veterinary profession lost an excellent clinician and research worker; it also lost an outstanding clinical teacher. Those of us who were fortunate to have been his pupils will long remember his patience and dedication as a teacher, for which the book will be a constant reminder.

During the revision of 'Ed's book' I have attempted to maintain his practical and clinically relevant style, whilst updating those areas in which new information has become available since 1988. The entire text has been revised and there are additional sections on the use of diagnostic ultrasound, the treatment of post-coital endometritis, diseases of the stallion, semen evaluation and the preservation of semen.

I am grateful to Mr John Newcombe BVetMed MRCVS for his comments on the first edition of the book, and for his advice during the preparation of the second edition.

I hope that this book continues to be a primary source of information as well as stimulating further study of equine reproduction.

G.C.W. England
1996

1 Anatomy of the Mare's Genital Tract

1.1 VULVA

- Lies below the anus (at risk from contamination by faeces).
- Normally almost vertical with firmly closed lips (Fig. 1.1.).
- Correct vulvar seal prevents pneumovagina.
- Three distinct vulvoperineal conformational types recognised.

1.2 VESTIBULE

- Extends from vulval lips to vestibulo-vaginal constriction.
- Has pink to brownish red mucous membrane.
- Ventrally houses the clitoris which is surrounded laterally and ventrally by clitoral fossa.
- May be palpated *per rectum*.

1.3 CLITORIS

- The dorsal surface of the clitoris contains up to three small cavities, the clitoral sinuses (**14.1**).
- Clitoral sinuses frequently covered by transverse frenular fold.
- Clitoral sinuses and fossae contain a variable amount of smegma.

1.4 VULVO-VAGINAL CONSTRICTION

- Just anterior to the external urethral opening.
- May be partial remnants or in maiden mares complete hymen at this junction.
- In genitally healthy mares this constriction forms a secondary line of defence against aspirated air and faecal material.

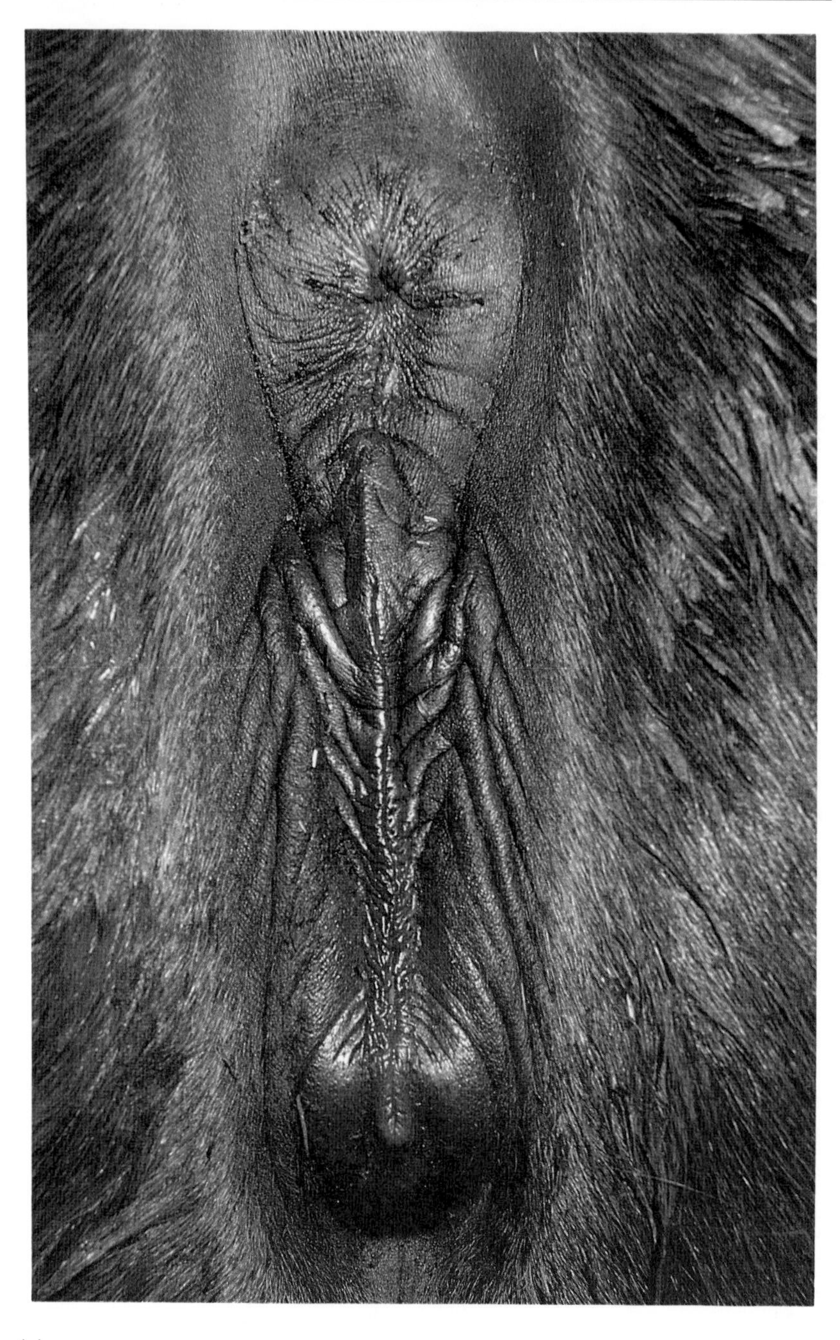

(a)

Fig. 1.1. Photographs of the perineal region of two mares.
(a) Normal conformation. The vulva is almost vertically orientated and the majority of the vulva is positioned ventral to the pelvic floor. This conformation results in establishment of a vulval seal preventing aspiration of air into the vagina. Additionally there will be little or no faecal contamination of the vulva during defaecation.

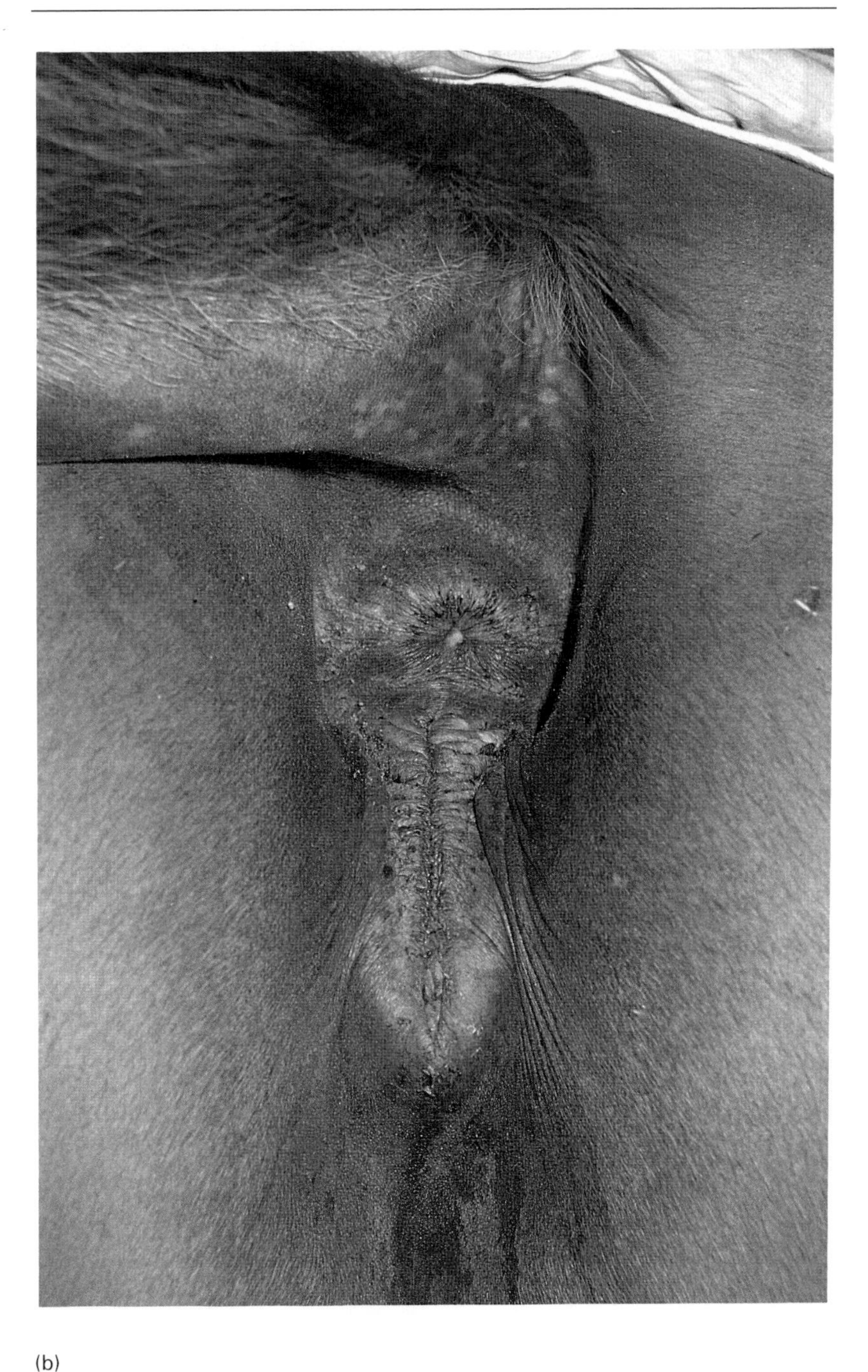

(b)

(b) Abnormal conformation. The anus is sunken causing the vulva to be pulled cranially. The dorsal vulva is almost horizontal in its orientation. This conformation results in absence of the normal vulval seal and air may be aspirated into the vagina. There will be significant contamination of the vulva with faeces at defaecation.

1.5 VAGINA

- A potentially hollow tube which when undisturbed is completely collapsed.
- Cyclical changes in the appearance of the vaginal mucosa are minimal.
- Most of the vagina is retroperitoneal.

1.6 CERVIX UTERI

- A tubular organ 4–10 cm long which protrudes into the cranial vagina.
- Last line of defence between uterine lumen and atmosphere.
- The length, diameter, tone and patency of the cervix varies greatly during different reproductive states (**4.1–4.9**).
- Part of the cervix projects caudally into the potential cavity of the vagina, and its appearance is useful for determining the mare's reproductive status.
- At no time in the normal mare is the cervix so tightly closed that it cannot be dilated manually.

1.7 UTERUS

- Roughly T or Y shaped in appearance and consists of a body and two horns (Fig. 1.2).
- Position may be changed by filling of the bladder or intestine.
- The body runs forward and downwards on the anterior floor of the pelvis, and caudal abdomen, dorsal, dorso-lateral or lateral to the bladder.
- The body averages 20 cm in length.
- The horns bifurcate from the cranial end of the body, and run laterally, or dorso-laterally.
- The horns average 20 to 25 cm in length.
- The horns are smaller in diameter at their tips.
- The normal non-pregnant uterus has a potential lumen.
- The thickness of the uterine walls, and the tone of the myometrium, vary with the reproductive state and age.
- Pregnancy causes gross distortion of the shape of the uterus (**7.1**).

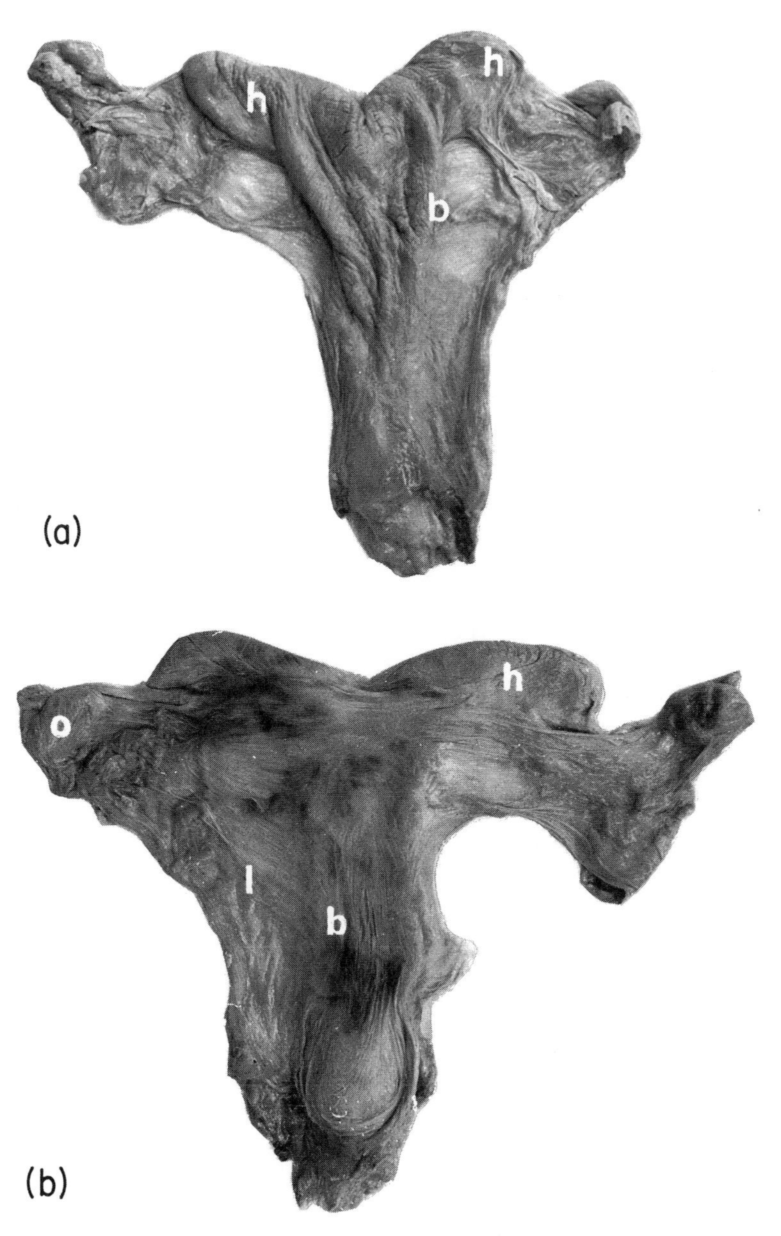

Fig. 1.2. (a) Ventral surface of uterus. (b) Dorsal surface of uterus. **h**, uterine horn; **b**, uterine body; **o**, ovary; **l**, broad ligament; **c**, cervix.

1.8 BROAD LIGAMENTS

- Each ligament extends from the dorso-caudal border of a horn, and the dorso-lateral border of the body to the sublumbar and lateral pelvic wall.
- Distal to the uterine horns they suspend, and expand to cover, the ovaries.
- Smooth muscle fibres within the broad ligament form the proper ligament of the ovary.

1.9 OVARIES

- Roughly bean shaped, but shape and size quite variable dependent mainly on follicular content (**4.1–4.9, 7.6**) (Fig. 1.3).
- Large variations in shape, size and consistency occur in normal mares.
- Anoestrus size ranges from 4 cm × 2 cm × 2 cm to 8 cm × 4 cm × 4 cm; tend to be largest in older and larger mares.
- Suspended in the antero-lateral part of the broad ligament (the mesovarium).
- The broad ligament between the ovary and tip of uterine horn is the tubal membrane (free margin of mesosalpinx).
- The ovary is covered by an extension of the broad ligament (serosa) except at the ovulation fossa, which is a marked depression on its antero-medial border.
- The uterine (Fallopian) tubes run within the tubal membrane.
- The amupulla of the uterine tube terminates in distinct fimbriae (infundibulum) positioned adjacent to the ovulation fossa between the proper ligament of the ovary and the tubal membrane.
- The uterine end of the uterine tube opens at the tip of the horn on a small papilla.

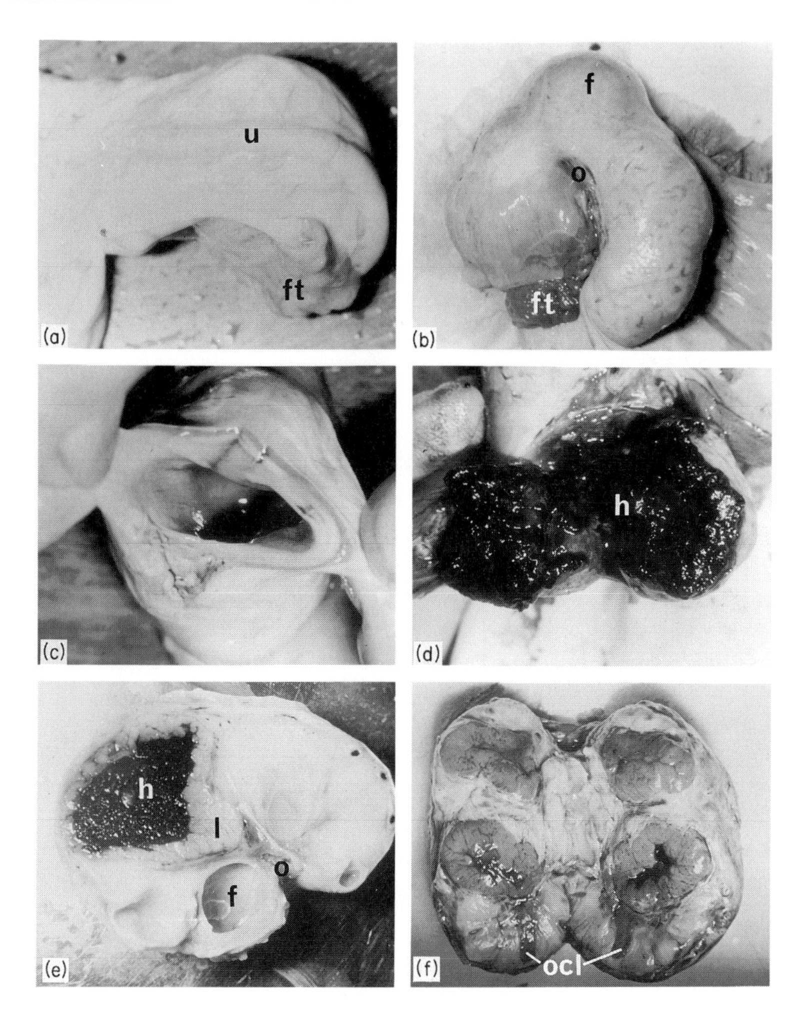

Fig. 1.3. (a) Lateral surface of ovary covered by mesosalpinx containing uterine tube. (b) Medial surface of ovary showing ovulation fossa. (c) Mature follicle opened to show fluid filled cavity. (d) Corpus haemorrhagicum sectioned to show extensive haematoma. (e) Formalin preserved ovary sectioned to show developing corpus luteum with central haematoma. (f) Sectioned ovary containing two mature corpora lutea, one of which has a central haematoma; the corpus luteum of the previous cycle has not yet turned yellow. **u**, uterine tube; **o**, ovulation fossa; **f**, follicle; **ft**, fimbriae of uterine tube; **h**, haematoma; **l**, luteal tissue; **ocl**, old corpus luteum.

2 Endocrinology of the Oestrous Cycle and Puberty

2.1 GENERAL

The mare is a seasonally polyoestrous breeder. Ovulation occurs spontaneously at the end of a variable follicular phase. The natural breeding season is May to October. Outside of the breeding season many (but not all) mares become anovulatory.

2.2 DEFINITIONS

Cycle length

This is the interval between two successive oestrous ovulations (but multiple ovulations during the same oestrus and dioestrous ovulations also occur). This is a more accurate measurement than the end of one heat to the end of the next. Cycle length is usually 21 ± 2 days but it is very variable. Longest cycle length occurs in spring. If cycle length is shorter than 18 days suspect endometritis (**13.1**). Abnormal persistence of the corpus luteum (**CL**) is called prolonged dioestrus, i.e. long cycle (**4.9**).

Anoestrus

Prolonged period of ovarian inactivity. Usually winter and spring, depending on mare and management system. Occasionally in summer, especially in lactating mares. May be small follicles up to 15 mm in ovaries. No functional CL.

Transitions from anoestrus to regular cycles (vernal transition)

Occurs in late winter or early spring, depending on mare and management. Variable follicular activity with many follicles, some reaching ovulatory size before becoming atretic; erratic oestrous behaviour. Oestrus behaviour may last more than a month before the first ovulation occurs.

Oestrus

Period of acceptance of the stallion. Usually lasts 4–7 days but very variable. Longest in spring (i.e. first heat of year); usually ends approximately 24 hours (0–48 hours) after ovulation. Under endocrine and psychological control. However, split-oestrus, silent heat and shy breeders may occur (**12.4, 12.5, 12.9**).

Interoestrus

Roughly synonymous with dioestrus, but more accurately describes the interval between two successive heats. Usually 14–16 days in length, but may be longer early in the year. May be short if CL lysed due to endometritis (**13.1**) or after prostaglandin (PG) administration (**5.2**). Prolonged due to persistence of the CL (prolonged dioestrus) (**4.9**).

Luteal phase

The time period between ovulation and luteolysis, i.e. 14 or 15 days. This may be shortened by endometritis or PG administration (after day 5). Short luteal phase may shorten the interoestrous period but not always, especially in spring. Long luteal phase occurs where corpus luteum is not lysed spontaneously and it may persist for up to three months (prolonged dioestrus).

2.3 HORMONAL CHANGES

The cycle is controlled by five major hormones (Fig. 2.1).

- Follicle stimulating hormone (FSH) from anterior pituitary gland. Peak blood concentrations in mid-dioestrus approximately 10 days before ovulation. This stimulates initial follicular growth (not usually palpable within the ovaries). Low concentrations of FSH are found during oestrus.
- Luteinising hormone (LH) from anterior pituitary gland. Circulating concentrations are low in the late luteal phase. Initial rise occurs in early oestrus and reaches peak values after ovulation. In the mare, this hormone stimulates major follicular growth, maturation and ovulation. Values decrease as progesterone concentrations (from the developing CL) rise.
- Progesterone. Secreted by corpus haemorrhagicum (**4.5**) and corpus luteum. Blood concentrations start to rise after ovulation and reach a peak 5 to 9 days later. During the first 4–5 days the developing CL is refractory to prostaglandin (**5.2**). High concentrations of progesterone maintained until day 14, when the CL is usually lysed by endogenous PG released from the uterus. CL persists spontaneously in prolonged dioestrus and pregnancy.
- Prostaglandin $F_2\alpha$ released from the endometrium. Released 13 to 15 days after ovulation under the action of oxytocin. Enters general circulation and if quantities reaching the CL are sufficient, causes luteolysis.

Endometritis and intrauterine manipulation during luteal phase cause premature PG release (**13.1**).

- Oestrogens. Secreted by the ovarian follicles. Oestradiol 17-β and conjugated oestrogens, especially oestrone sulphate. Concentrations low during most of cycle but rise in early oestrus to reach peak values 48 hours before ovulation.

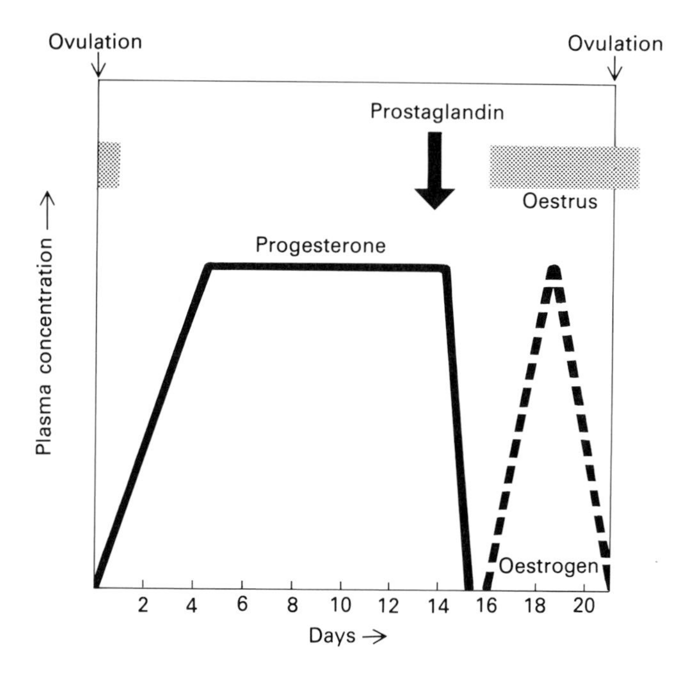

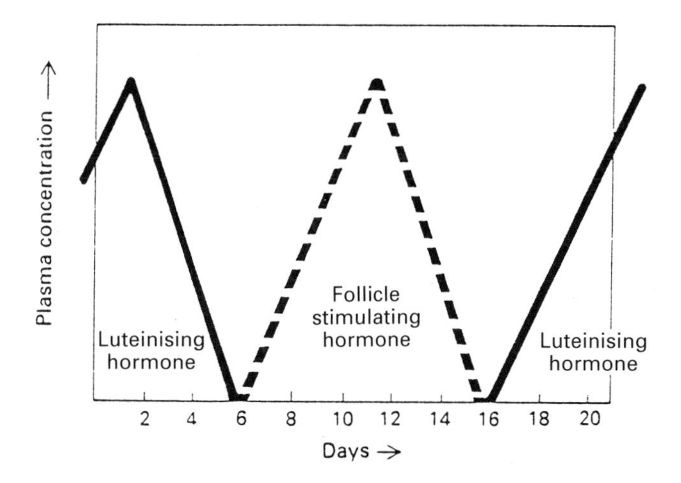

Fig. 2.1. Diagrammatic representation of the major hormonal events in the mare's oestrous cycle.

2.4 PUBERTY

Usually reached by 2 years of age, but some mares may ovulate as yearlings in late summer especially if born early in the year. Puberty delayed by poor nutrition, being in training, and/or the administration of anabolic steroids. Turner's syndrome (XO – sex chromosome aneuploidy) may be mistaken for immaturity. Similarly young mares in deep anoestrus may appear to be pre-pubertal.

3 Clinical Examination of the Mare's Genital Tract

Basic examination of the genital tract consists of:

- visual examination of the perineum, vulva and tail
- manual palpation of the cervix, uterus and ovaries *per rectum*
- visual inspection of the vagina and cervix *per vaginam* using a speculum
- manual palpation of the vagina and cervix *per vaginam*
- real time ultrasound imaging *per rectum* (for other methods of examination see **11.3**).

3.1 RESTRAINT OF THE MARE

- Amount of restraint needed depends on experience, and temperament of mare, and quality and quantity of help available. Examination is most difficult in young undisciplined mares handled by amateurs, and easiest in old brood mares handled by experienced personnel. The presence of a foal at foot may make examination of mares more difficult. No method of restraint is ideal.
- Temperament of mare. Some mares are vicious and kick when handled behind; these are uncommon. Most mares are apprehensive when examined for the first time and may need more restraint than subsequently. Most mares tend to walk forward or move sideways if only loosely restrained during examination. The presence (or absence) of the mare's foal, or separation from a companion may make the mare uneasy, as can the sight of unfamiliar objects (clinician's protective clothing, coloured sleeves, lubricant bottles, etc.). Examining mares in a field is made more difficult and more dangerous by the presence of other inquisitive horses.

Stocks

Probably the best method of restraint but:

- mare may not enter easily, especially for first time
- mare may be uneasy about being confined, especially initially
- mare may try to jump out, especially to join a companion or foal (it may

be possible to put the foal in the stocks with the mare, otherwise the foal is best placed directly in front of the stocks)
- ensure that the back panel of the stocks is low
- stocks should be readily dismantleable as occasionally mares become cast.

Twitch

Very useful method of restraint and may be only form necessary for most mares, but:

- some owners resent the application of a twitch to their mare
- some mares are very difficult to twitch
- some mares won't move when twitched, so position correctly beforehand
- some mares try to go down when twitched tightly
- twitch will not always control a wilful mare
- humane twitch (Fig. 3.1) is easy to apply and leaves no mark on the nose. Not suitable for ponies (nose is too small).

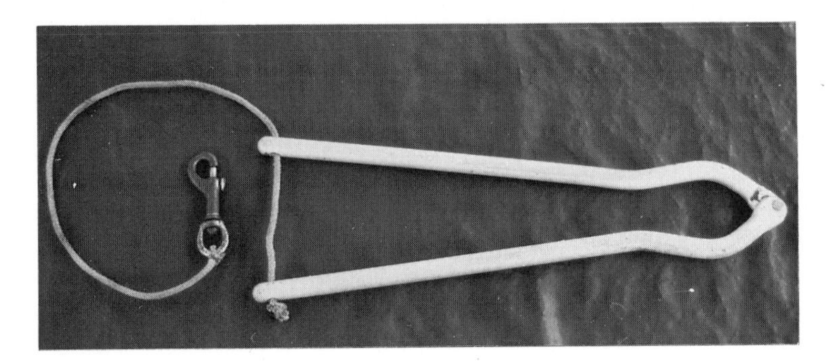

Fig. 3.1. Humane twitch.

Bridle

May be used with twitch or other methods. Helps the handler to stop the mare moving forward; a chiffney bit gives best control.

Bales

Bales of hay or straw behind the mare give some degree of protection against kicks, but:

- mare may resent presence of bales
- mare may take a step forward during initial examination.

Other methods of restraint

Lifting a front leg, on the side of the examiner, stops the mare from kicking with the ipsilateral back leg, but:

- the clinician may have to stand directly behind the mare
- the back end of the mare tends to be lowered, which makes rectal examination particularly difficult
- an inexperienced helper may suddenly release the forelimb, or take too much of the mare's weight so that she can still kick.

Turning the mare's head towards the examiner helps to prevent her kicking with the hind leg on that same side.

Hind-leg hobbles help to prevent kicking but are seldom used in the UK.

Low doses of the α_2-adrenoceptor agonists (detomidine, romifidine, xylazine) may be useful; especially since they are anxiolytic.

3.2 APPROACH OF THE CLINICIAN

Avoid sudden movements and loud noises, but try to converse with helper in an even voice, or hum or whistle.

When mare is not in stocks, approach her from the side, put one hand on the back, run it to base of the tail, grasp tail and pull it to one side.

- At this stage, mare's temperament and effectiveness of restraint will become apparent.
- Feel for discharge (wet or dried) on tail, and inspect perineum (**13.1, 15.5**).
- For manual examination *per rectum* or *vaginam*, the arm can be inserted initially without the operator standing directly behind the mare. As examination proceeds, more the clinician's body is behind the mare, but at this stage her likely reaction has been anticipated.
- For speculum examination *per vaginam*, it is most convenient for an assistant to hold the tail (in a gloved hand) to allow the clinician a free hand to part the vulval lips.

Round the door-post approach, with the mare against the wall. This is not advisable as:

- mare may resent initial positioning
- if mare steps forward during initial examination, clinician becomes exposed.

Examination over half-door not recommended except for clitoral swabbing (**14.1**); they are usually far too high.

Standing mare in a doorway with the back half in the yard is ideal for quiet mares (with or without twitch) which are accustomed to being examined. A light outside the box aids in speculum examination, and standing outside the box may protect ultrasound equipment although the ultrasound screen is more difficult to visualise. It may be difficult to persuade the mare to stop halfway through the doorway.

3.3 EXTERNAL EXAMINATION

This may reveal:

- Normal vulva – nearly perpendicular, no distortions (scarring) or discharges.
- Sunken anus (due to old age, poor condition) common in Thoroughbreds and causes antero-dorsal displacement of dorsal commisure of the vulva. This encourages contamination of the vulva and vestibule with faeces and predisposes to pneumovagina (**13.2**).
- Vulva already sutured (Caslick's operation) to prevent pneumovagina.
- Lateral or dorsal tears to vulva.
- Small vesicles or ulcerated areas due to coital exanthema (herpesvirus 3 – **16.2**). Not to be confused with small depigmented areas which are common.
- Vulval discharge. Varies from sticky moistness at ventral commisure to frank discharge (wet or dried) on thighs and tail (**13.1**). A small amount of moisture is normal during oestrus, especially after covering, when a temporary purulent discharge may be seen.
- Yellow urine stain (usually dry) on ventral commisure of vulva. Usually denotes oestrus (but not always present) – due to increased urinary frequency when showing (winking) (**4.3**).

3.4 MANUAL EXAMINATION *per rectum*

- Due to the lateral position of the ovaries, one-handed rectal examination makes accurate palpation of the right ovary for the right-handed examiner (and vice versa) difficult if the mare is not well restrained.
- Wear a glove and use adequate lubricant.
- Mare usually resents passage of hand most and then the elbow.
- Evacuate rectum of faeces totally and feel for uterine horns lying transversely in front of the pubis. Follow these laterally to ovaries which are cranial to the shaft of ileum.
- Always try to have hand cranial to the structure which is to be palpated to allow sufficient rectum for manipulation.
- Do not stretch rectum laterally if tense; do not resist strong peristaltic contractions – otherwise rectum may tear (especially dorsally, i.e. not adjacent to examiner's hand) (**28.4**).
- If the rectum is ballooned with air, feel forward for peristaltic constriction and gently stroke with a finger to stimulate contraction.
- Ovaries often lie lateral to broad ligament and are difficult to palpate. They must be manipulated onto the cranio-medial aspect of the ligament for accurate palpation.
- Uterus is very difficult to palpate in anoestrus, easier during cycles, and easiest during early (up to 60 days) pregnancy, due to increasing thickness and tone of the uterine wall (**4.1, 4.3, 7.1**).

- Cervix is palpated by sweeping fingertips ventrally from side to side in mid pelvic area. It is easiest to feel during the luteal phase, but more difficult during oestrus and anoestrus (**4.1, 4.3, 4.6**).

3.5 VISUAL EXAMINATION *per vaginam*

- Requires optimal restraint, as operator will have to stand behind the mare.
- Clean perineum and vulva with clean water or weak disinfectant.
- Moisten or lubricate speculum.
- After introducing speculum through vulval lips, push cranio-dorsally to clear brim of pubis.
- At this point there is often considerable resistance at vestibulo-vaginal junction (occasionally the speculum tries to enter the urethra).
- When fully inserted (±30 cm) view vaginal walls and cervix.
- Make evaluation quickly because artifactual reddening can occur following contact with speculum or air onto vaginal wall.

Types of speculum (see also uterine swabbing, **14.2**)

1. *Metal*, e.g. Russian duck-billed. Good visualisation but cumbersome and difficult to clean. It requires a separate light source which must be protected.
2. *Plastic*. Replaceable tubular speculum with integral light source. If vagina does not balloon with air, cervix is difficult to visualise. Reduces likelihood of spreading venereal infection. Difficult to visualise dorsal wall of vagina (e.g. for recto-vaginal fistula, **13.2**). Light source often temperamental.
3. *Cardboard*. Tubular with silvered interior to reflect light. Requires separate light source. Slightly longer than plastic speculum but disposable and cheap – avoids resterilisation.

3.6 MANUAL EXAMINATION *per vaginam*

- Clean vulva and insert lubricated gloved hand.
- May feel remnants of hymen – occasionally complete (**12.16**).
- Vagina dry in luteal phase and anoestrus, moist in oestrus, sticky mucus in pregnancy.
- Palpate cervix for shape, size and patency of canal.
- May detect adhesions or fibrosis (**12.15**).
- Do not force finger along cervical canal if there is a possibility of pregnancy.
- Mare's cervix will allow gentle dilation without causing damage, at all stages of reproduction.

- Manual examination may not be possible if mare's vulva is sutured excessively tightly (**13.2**).

3.7 ULTRASOUND EXAMINATION *per rectum*

Principles of diagnostic ultrasound

- Diagnostic ultrasound utilises sound frequencies between 2 and 10 MHz.
- Ultrasound is produced by application of an alternating voltage to piezoelectric crystals which change in size and produce a pressure or ultrasound wave. Returning echoes deform the same crystals which generate a surface voltage.
- Most diagnostic ultrasound machines use the principle of brightness modulation (B-mode) where the returning echoes are displayed as dots, the brightness of which is proportional to their amplitude.
- Real-time B-mode ultrasound is a dynamic imaging system where information is continually updated and displayed on a monitor.
- Ultrasound is attenuated within tissues and attenuation is related to wavelength of the sound, the density of the tissue, the heterogeneity of the tissue and the number and type of echo interfaces.
- Bright (specular) echoes are produced when a large proportion of the beam is reflected back to the transducer; these echoes are displayed as white areas on the ultrasound machine screen.
- No echoes are produced when the sound is transmitted and not reflected; these areas are displayed as black on the ultrasound machine screen.
- Non-specular echoes are produced when the beam encounters a structure similar to one wavelength in size, and these echoes appear as varying shades of grey on the ultrasound machine screen.

The ultrasound transducer

- Piezoelectric crystals are arranged together to form an ultrasound transducer, contained within the ultrasound head.
- The crystals may be arranged:
    in a line (linear array transducer)
    in an arc (sector transducer)
    in an arc and electronically triggered (phased array transducer)
    mounted upon a rotating wheel (mechanical sector transducer).
- Transducers produce sound of a characteristic frequency.
    High frequencies allow good resolution although there is greater attenuation of the sound beam in tissues.
    Low frequencies allow a greater depth of penetration (less attenuation) but with reduced resolution.

Equipment for examination of the mare

- Linear array transducers are most suited to transrectal imaging.
- Linear array transducers allow a large field of view in the near field and are generally robust.
- For the examination of ovarian structures and of early pregnancy a 7.5 MHz transducer is most suitable.
- For the examination of late pregnancy a 3.5 MHz transducer is necessary.
- A 5.0 MHz transducer offers a compromise which gives a reasonable depth of penetration combined with adequate tissue resolution.
- The ultrasound machine should be small and lightweight, have a keyboard to allow identification of the animal and possess electronic callipers to allow measurement of images.
- There should be facilities to record the images and this can be achieved using:
  - a thermal printer
  - a Polaroid camera
  - a multiformat camera.

Ultrasound terminology

- Tissues that markedly reflect sound (such as gas, bone and metal) appear white on the ultrasound screen and are called echogenic.
- Tissues that transmit sound (such as fluid) appear black on the ultrasound screen and are called anechogenic (or anechoic).
- Tissues that allow some transmission and some reflection (such as most soft tissues) appear as varying shades of grey and are called hypoechogenic or hyperechogenic depending upon their exact appearance.
- Strictly a hyperechogenic tissue produces a hyperechoic region within the image, although these terms are often used synonymously.

Examination of the mare

- Safety is paramount and mares are ideally restrained in suitable stocks.
- Foals are best positioned either in front of the stocks or within the stocks adjacent to the mare.
- The rectum should be emptied of faecal material to ensure a good contact between the transducer and the rectal wall. Attempts to manipulate the transducer when the rectum is filled with faecal material may result in tearing of the rectal wall.
- Should the mare strain during the examination the transducer should be withdrawn.

Imaging technique

- The examination should be performed out of direct sunlight since this can hinder interpretation of images on the ultrasound screen.

- The ultrasound transducer is usually held within the rectum in the sagittal (longitudinal) plane during imaging.
- The vestibule and vagina lie within the pelvis in the midline; these structures can be imaged with ultrasound but are indistinct.
- The cervix is located cranial to the vagina approximately 20 cm cranial to the anal sphincter and can be identified as a heterogeneous, generally hyperechogenic, region with a rectangular outline.
- The uterus is roughly 'T' or 'Y' shaped; therefore when using a linear ultrasound transducer the outline of the uterine body generally appears rectangular (the transducer is in a sagittal plane) whilst the outline of the uterine horns appears circular (the transducer whilst orientated in the sagittal plane is positioned in a transverse plane with respect to the uterine horn) (Fig. 3.2).
- The uterus has a central homogeneous, relatively hypoechoic, region surrounded by a peripheral hyperechoic layer.
- The echogenicity of the endometrium and the uterine cross sectional diameter vary during the oestrous cycle; during oestrus the diameter increases and the uterus becomes increasingly hypoechoic with central radiating hyperechoic lines which are typical of endometrial oedema.
- The proximal uterine horns are of smaller diameter than the uterine body.
- The ovaries can be located by tracing the uterine horns laterally.
- Various sections of the ovaries are usually examined by rotation of the transducer; sections are usually taken from a medial position, and sequential sections of the ventral, mid, and dorsal portions of the ovaries are examined.
- Ovaries usually contain follicles (which are anechoic), and may contain luteal structures (which are relatively echogenic – varying shades of grey-white); the ovarian stroma may be difficult to appreciate since it may be surrounded by these structures although it is generally hypoechoic in appearance.

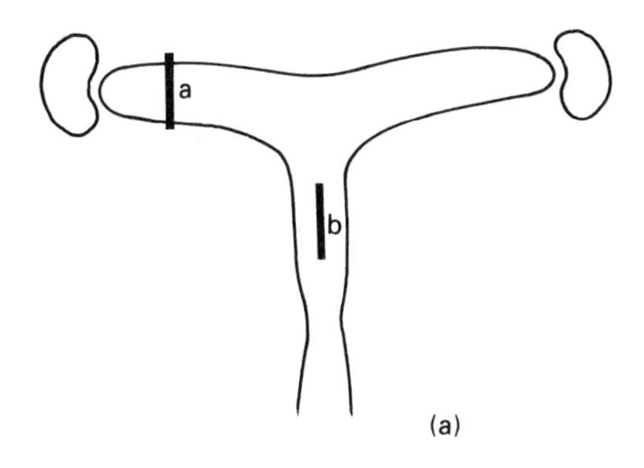

(a)

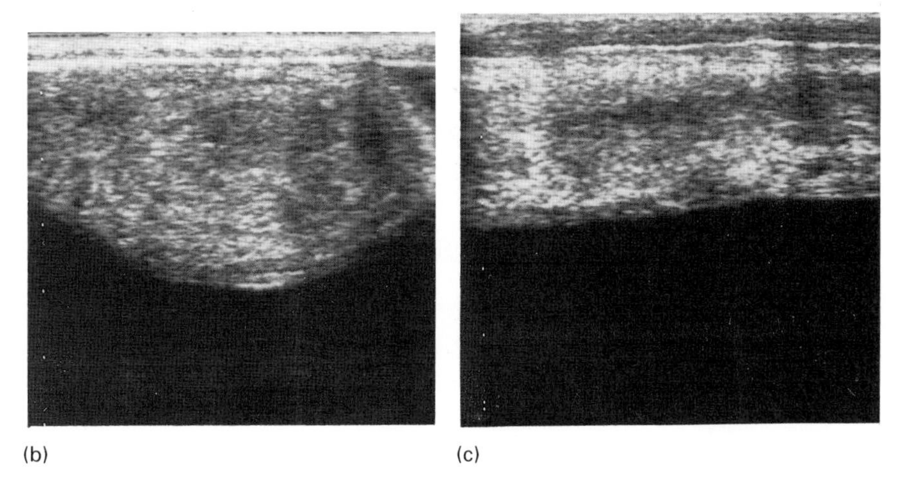

(b)

(c)

Fig. 3.2.
(a) Schematic representation of the uterus of a non-pregnant mare demonstrating the position of the ultrasound transducer in relation to the uterine horn (a), and uterine body (b). (b) Ultrasound image of the uterine horn positioned dorsal to the bladder – transverse section (7.5 MHz transducer, scale in cm). (c) Ultrasound image of the uterine body positioned dorsal to the bladder – sagittal section (7.5 MHz transducer, scale in cm).

4 Cyclical Changes in the Mare's Genital Tract

4.1 ANOESTRUS

Rectal palpation

- Ovaries: small, hard, bean shaped, may have small follicles.
- Uterus: thin walled and flaccid, may be difficult to palpate.
- Cervix: soft and indistinct.

Visual examination of the vagina

- Vaginal wall is pale (blanched) and dry.
- Cervix is flaccid and atonic; closed but may gape open to reveal uterine lumen.

Palpation *per vaginam*

- Vagina is dry.
- Cervix is dry, short and easily admits two fingers but may be tighter in maiden and older mares.

Ultrasound examination (Fig. 4.1)

- Ovaries: small, multiple small follicles (less than 1.5 cm diameter) no luteal tissue.
- Uterus: small, homogeneous hypoechoic appearance.

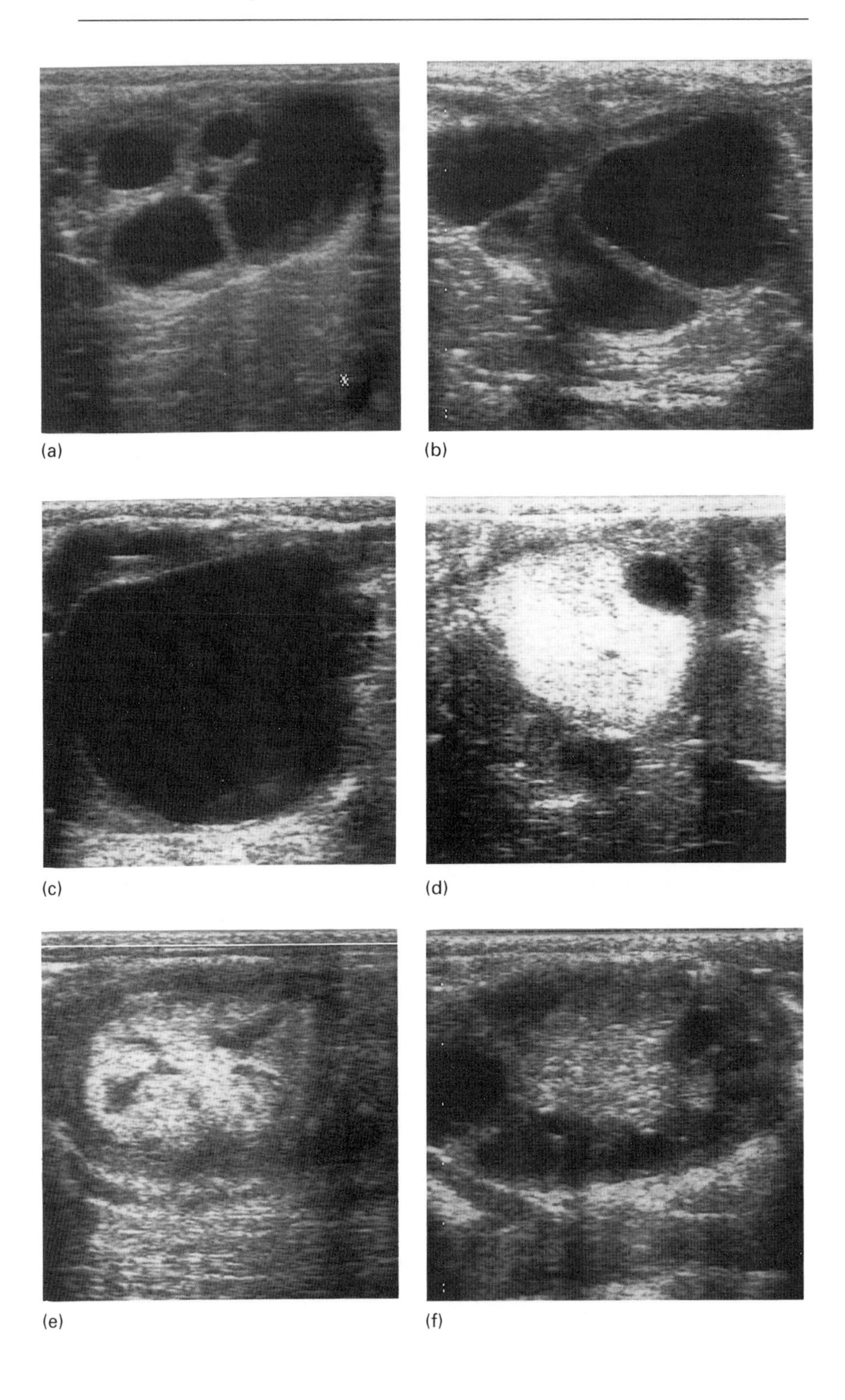
(a)
(b)
(c)
(d)
(e)
(f)

4.2 TRANSITION

Rectal palpation

- Ovaries: become softer, follicles grow (3–5 cm) and then regress. May be repeated waves of follicular growth and regression. Difficult to anticipate which follicle will grow and when. Ovulation usually followed by regular ovulatory cycles.
- Uterus: flaccid or slight tone, may be similar to oestrus.
- Cervix: remains soft and difficult to palpate *per rectum*.

Visual examination of the vagina

- Vaginal wall appearance depends upon ovarian function, i.e. from typically anoestrus to typically oestrus.
- Cervix frequently appears similar to early oestrus (below).

Paplation *per vaginam*

- Vagina and cervix frequently feel similar to early oestrus (below).

Fig. 4.1. Ultrasound images of ovaries at various stages of the oestrous cycle (7.5 MHz transducer, scale in cm).
(a) Late anoestrus. Four small anechoic follicles are present within the ovary. The ovarian stroma can be seen between the follicles, and is relatively hypoechoic in appearance. (b) Oestrus. One medium-sized follicle predominates; however, several smaller follicles are present peripherally. It is likely that the larger follicle has been recruited and will ovulate.
(c) Preovulatory. A single large, soft preovulatory follicle is present; the time of ovulation may be anticipated by the size, shape and echogenicity of the follicle. (d) Post-ovulation. The follicular cavity has been filled with blood clot and has become markedly echoic in appearance. This early luteal structure may be termed a corpus haemorrhagicum (CH), although it is correct to refer to it as a corpus luteum. Not all CHs are entirely echogenic and some may have fluid filled cavities within them. (e) Ageing of the CH results in a decrease in its echogenicity and a reduction in its size. In this example, three days after ovulation, the structure was still palpable *per rectum*. This structure is not homogeneous and has several hypoechoic zones which may be luteal tissue, or areas of fluid accumulation.
(f) Dioestrus. A well-delineated corpus luteum with a homogeneous hypoechoic appearance is present within the ovary. Small anechoic follicles are present in a peripheral position.

Ultrasound examination

- Ovaries: large, contain multiple follicles of varying sizes. In early transition follicles may be multiple and small; later follicular size increases and follicles may reach 5 cm in diameter. Follicles regress (decrease in size) without ovulating. No luteal tissue is identified.
- Uterus: frequently oedema (see below) present, associated with growth of a specific follicle. Oedema is more variable than during oestrus of the normal breeding season. Anechoic (black) free luminal fluid may be present.

4.3 OESTRUS

Rectal palpation

- Ovaries: follicles 2–3 cm diameter identified on the first day. One or more grow to 3–6 cm before ovulation. Sometimes follicles may be less than this size (3 cm) at ovulation. Distinct follicular softening may be detected as ovulation approaches.
- Uterus: endometrial folds enlarge and become oedematous. Uterus feels thickened, heavier and 'doughy' but not tonic (cf. cow).
- Cervix: feels soft and broad when fully relaxed. In some mares it may be soft cranially and firmer caudally. Usually shorter than during dioestrus.

Visual examination of the vagina

- The vulva may relax during oestrus, although this is not consistent. Sometimes a slight mucoid discharge or yellow stain is noted on the ventral vulval commissure due to frequent urination.
- The vaginal wall appearance changes through pink, bright pink to red as oestrus progresses.
- Increasing moistness with decreasing viscosity.
- Cervix progressively flattens and sinks to the vaginal floor.
- Cervical os appears as a horizontal slit.
- Appearance similar to a 'wilted rose'.

Palpation *per vaginam*

- Vagina is moist.
- Cervix is obviously soft and oedematous, and admits one to three fingers as oestrus progresses.
- Cervix may be more dilated at the foal heat.
- Cervix may contract when palpated.

Ultrasound examination

- Ovaries: large, between one and three follicles predominate and protrude above ovarian margin. Follicles appear flattened (margin adjacent to transducer becomes flat) as softening occurs. Corpora lutea of previous cycle may still be evident as triangular echogenic region. Follicle wall increases in thickness and echogenicity as ovulation approaches. Follicle may assume triangular outline as it 'points' towards the ovulation fossa (ovulation does not occur over the surface of the ovary only at the ovulation fossa).

- Uterus: increases in diameter commencing early oestrus. Endometrium becomes oedematous and individual endometrial folds can be seen. Folds appear as intertwining areas of hyper- and hypoechogenicity. Hypoechogenic regions are the result of submucosal fluid (oedema). The degree of uterine oedema increases with follicle growth. Oedema generally reduces commencing one day prior to ovulation, but this is not always the case. Free luminal fluid may occasionally be seen. In the normal mare this fluid is anechoic.

4.4 OVULATION

Accurate detection can only be achieved by daily examination of the mare. Ovulation always occurs at the ovulation fossa (Fig. 1.2). During ovulation follicular fluid and the oocyte are released (fimbriae of the infundibulum cover the ovulation fossa at this time to collect the oocyte). After ovulation the follicle is collapsed, but refills with blood within approximately 12 hours. This structure may be termed a corpus haemorrhagicum (CH). Gradual luteinisation of this structure results in the formation of a corpus luteum (CL).

Accurate detection of ovulation is important because it:

- confirms that ovulation has occurred
- confirms time of ovulation in relation to service or insemination
- identifies multiple ovulations.

Rectal palpation

- Ovaries: mature follicles are generally large (>4 cm) and soft, and just before ovulation may become very soft and tender. Occasionally follicles collapse during palpation of the ovary – this does not affect fertility; it is difficult and inadvisable to try to rupture follicles manually. At ovulation follicular fluid is expelled and the wall of the follicle collapses. The surface of the ovary may be depressed in this region. The follicular cavity, however, rapidly fills with blood and approximately 12 hours after ovulation the cavity is redistended. This corpus haemorrhagicum is usually about 80% of the diameter of the preovulatory follicle. It may have a similar texture to a preovulatory follicle, and ovulation detection may be difficult if the examination interval is more than 24 hours. The CH may be similar sized to, or larger than, the preovulatory follicle. In either case it functions as a normal CH/CL. At ovulation the ovary is often tender when palpated (mare twitches her flank, looks at flank, or kicks at belly).

- Uterus and cervix: there are no specific changes in these structures at the time of ovulation; they demonstrate typical oestrous characteristics.

Visual examination of the vagina

- Vaginal wall is moist and hyperaemic, but there are no specific changes associated with ovulation.

Palpation *per vaginam*

- Vagina is moist and cervix is soft and oedematous, but there are no specific changes associated with ovulation.

Ultrasound examination

- Ovaries: preceding ovulation the follicle may be seen to flatten (indicating softening) and 'point' towards the ovulation fossa. Ovulation is detected by the disappearance of the large fluid filled (anechoic) follicle. Two evacuation patterns have been described, although it is likely that such simple classifications are not accurate. During evacuation follicle diameter decreases, and the follicle wall becomes irregular. Detection of the empty follicular cavity can be difficult. Fortunately in many cases a small volume of fluid remains within the cavity. Redistention of the follicular cavity with blood is readily detected with ultrasound. The central clot appears markedly echogenic (bright white) in appearance. Central residual fluid may still be present.
- Uterus: generally the degree of endometrial oedema and the amount of luminal fluid decrease prior to ovulation, although this is not always the case.

4.5 DEVELOPMENT OF THE CORPUS LUTEUM

Luteinisation begins immediately after ovulation. Plasma progesterone concentrations are elevated earlier than most domestic species.

Development of the mature corpus luteum from the corpus haemorrhagicum is a gradual process which takes 4–6 days. The maturing corpus luteum becomes smaller and firmer due to:

- shrinkage of the thrombus, which is also being invaded by:
- rapidly dividing peripheral (thecal) cells which become luteal cells (and produce progesterone), and
- condensation of the ovarian stroma which becomes thicker around the CL due to its diminished surface area.

Rectal palpation

- Ovaries: the early CH/CL may be palpable, and feel similar to a pre-ovulatory follicle. Later the structure becomes firmer and smaller in diameter. The CL is usually not palpable from 4–5 days after ovulation. Presence of the CL may be suggested by enlargement of one pole of the ovary (although the luteal structure itself cannot be palpated). CLs which result from large CHs remain palpable for a longer period of time.
- Uterus: reduces in diameter; uterine oedema (therefore 'doughy' texture) is lost. Uterus feels more tonic.
- Cervix: reduces in diameter and increases in tone.

Visual examination of the vagina

- Vaginal wall starts to become pale and dry.
- Cervix becomes grey and cervical os becomes contracted.

Palpation *per vaginam*

- Vagina is dry.
- Cervix is dry with increased tone and cervical os becomes closed.

Ultrasound examination

- Ovaries: the corpus haemorrhagicum is generally hyperechogenic in appearance. It may or may not have a central fluid filled (anechoic) region. The relative size of any central anechoic region tends to decrease after day 3. After this time as the CL ages it tends to reduce in diameter and in echogenicity.
- Uterus: endometrial oedema is normally absent. In the normal mare there is no luminal fluid.

4.6 DIOESTRUS (INTEROESTRUS)

From approximately five days after ovulation the luteal structure is mature. Progesterone concentrations have reached a high plateau. The CL now responds to exogenous prostaglandins.

Endogenous prostaglandins are produced from the endometrium on days 13–15.

Rectal palpation

- Ovaries: CL generally becomes less palpable. One ovary (containing CL) often larger than the other. Follicles may be present during the luteal phase (after mid luteal rise in FSH). Rarely dioestrous ovulations occur (cervix remains closed and tonic, and progesterone concentrations remain high).

- Uterus: becomes more tonic (tubular) especially in the late luteal phase. Uterine changes are not palpably consistent and vary greatly among mares.
- Cervix: firm and tubular. Approximately 8 cm in length, and 1 cm in width.

Visual examination of the vagina

- Vaginal wall dull white/yellow grey.
- Cervix becomes prominent and protruding, grey in colour.
- Cervical os is tight and centrally located; 'rose bud' appearance.

Palpation *per vaginam*

- Vagina is dry, viscous fluids, vaginal walls stick together.
- Cervix is dry, firm and protruding.
- Difficult to locate cervical os. (NB: Normal mare's cervix will always dilate to accommodate a finger, even during pregnancy).

Ultrasound examination

- Ovaries: size may depend upon season of the year. Moderately echogenic CL can always be identified. CL is often slightly triangular in shape (apex directed towards the ovulation fossa), with central line of echogenic tissue. Follicular growth may be present (more common in late luteal phase); large follicles may be evident.
- Uterus: small in diameter compared with oestrus. Endometrium has no oedema (homogeneous echotexture); location of the lumen may be identifiable by the presence of a small white line. Luminal fluid, if present, is abnormal.

4.7 LATE DIOESTRUS COMPARED WITH EARLY OESTRUS

In the normal mare endogenous prostaglandin results in lysis of the CL and a rapid return to oestrus. It may not be possible to distinguish between these two phases. Palpation and visual inspection reveal a state mid way between dioestrus and oestrus.

Rectal palpation

- Ovaries: the CL is not palpable, although its presence may be suggested by enlargement of one pole of the ovary. Follicles of varying size may be present in late dioestrus and early oestrus.
- Uterus: increases in diameter, uterine oedema may start to develop as oestrogen concentrations increase.
- Cervix: increases in diameter and becomes less tonic.

Visual examination of the vagina

- Vaginal wall starts to become moist and hyperaemic.
- Cervix becomes moist and cervical os becomes relaxed.

Palpation *per vaginam*

- Vagina is less dry.
- Cervix is moist with decreased tone and cervical os becomes relaxed.

Ultrasound examination

- Ovaries: the CL is usually visible as a small hypoechogenic structure. Follicular growth predominates. One or more follicles may have been recruited to ovulate at the next oestrus.
- Uterus: minor endometrial oedema may be present.

4.8 EARLY DIOESTRUS COMPARED WITH EARLY OESTRUS

It may be difficult to distinguish between these two phases of the cycle without ultrasonographic examination.

- The cervix takes 2–4 days to change from oestrous to luteal and vice versa.
- Uterine size and tone are similarly not diagnostic.
- Follicles and CH/CLs may be difficult to distinguish without ultrasound imaging.
- Mare shows similar behavioural responses to stallion.
- Ultrasound examination will demonstrate:
  presence of an echogenic CH in early dioestrus
  presence of follicles and an aged CL in early oestrus.

4.9 PROLONGED LUTEAL PHASE

An important cause of infertility. Persistence of the CL may be due to:

- idiopathic persistence of the CL
- failure of CL to respond to PG because of dioestrus ovulation
- inability of the uterus to secrete PG (uterine damage e.g. pyometra)
- foetal inhibition of PG secretion (pregnancy or pseudopregnancy)
- pharmacological inhibition of PG secretion.

Clinical features

- Ovaries: CL not palpable but can be imaged with ultrasound. Follicles usually present; can be multiple and large (3–5 cm). Increasing number and size with increased length of dioestrus. Some of these follicles ovulate despite the high concentrations of progesterone.

- Uterus: usually tubular and tonic, with no oedema. Features not discernible from late luteal phase or early pregnancy.
- Cervix: similar to late luteal phase or early pregnancy.

5 Manipulation of Cyclical Activity

5.1 TO SHORTEN THE TRANSITION BETWEEN ANOESTRUS AND CYCLICAL ACTIVITY

The natural breeding season occurs in late spring or summer; however, modern horse breeding requires that foals are born in January. Mares must therefore conceive early in the year (outside of the normal breeding season).

The aim is to produce an ovulatory oestrus during mid February. In general it is difficult truly to shorten the transitional period; therefore its onset must be hastened by providing artificial light and increased nutrition during winter. Progestogens may be used once some follicular development (follicles greater than 2.5 cm in diameter) is evident. Progestogens may be administered either as oral formulations to be placed in the feed (altrenogest), or as intravaginal devices (progesterone ± oestradiol benzoate), although the latter are not presently licensed for use in the mare. Progestogens are generally administered for 10–16 days. In those cases when intensive management is not possible it may simply be best to delay breeding until April.

- Plan ahead.
- Provide light for a minimum of 16 hours daily, e.g. 7 AM–11 PM – alternatively leave lights on all night.
- Good quality light, i.e. 150 watt *clear* bulb in centre of 4 metre × 4 metre box or 1.3 metre (40 watt) strip light is essential.
- Ideally there should be light falling upon the eyes wherever the horse stands – avoid shadows cast by beams or partitions; high dark ceilings reflect very little light.
- It should be easy to read a newspaper wherever you stand in the box.
- If the light intensity is insufficient there is no response.
- Mares commencing the lighting regime in poor bodily condition take longer to respond than those in good condition; the aim is to increase the level of nutrition and consequently the mare's condition.
- It is just as important to ensure that mares already in good or fat condition are sufficiently well fed to maintain their body weight.

- The length of time taken from beginning the regime to ovulation (response time) is affected by several factors:

  (1) Initial condition of mare and rate of improvement.
  (2) Time of year – regime started early March probably 'works' about 2 weeks faster than if started in December/January.
  (3) Individual mare variation – occasionally mares are very slow to respond whilst others begin spontaneous ovulation several weeks earlier than would be expected.

- Growth of large follicles may be stimulated by the administration of progestogens.
- Progestogen therapy should be withdrawn when follicles have reached preovulatory size.
- The stage at which the course of treatment is started is relatively critical:

  (1) If started in deep anoestrus with no pre-lighting, the mare will remain anoestrus.
  (2) If started in shallow anoestrus with insufficient pre-lighting, the mare will come into season with follicular growth but without ovulation and will then return to anoestrus.
  (3) If started in shallow anoestrus, after 4–6 weeks of 'lights' or in prolonged oestrus in late March or early April then ovulation should result.
  (4) If started in prolonged oestrus from January to March without pre-lighting then ovulation will probably not occur.
  (5) If started in prolonged oestrus mid-April or later then the first ovulation could have occurred earlier without treatment.

- It appears that those mares which fail to ovulate after progestogen treatment return to a deeper anoestrus than might be expected, so that eventual ovulation, whether spontaneous or following another course, is later than would have otherwise occurred.
- Ovulation occurs 'classically' around 10 days after the last dose of progestogen, but this interval is very variable. Some mares enter prolonged oestrus, eventually ovulating after 3 or 4 weeks.
- Treatment starting in January and February often results in ovulation about 15 days after the last dose.
- Treatment given in April may result in ovulation within 7 days, but if a large follicle was present at the beginning of the course it may:

  (1) ovulate during the course
  (2) ovulate within 24–48 hours of the end of the course (with or without oestrus)
  (3) regress.

- Occasionally a small follicle may grow during progestogen treatment and then ovulate within 24–48 hours of the end.

- For all these reasons it is advisable to examine the mare on or about the last day of treatment.
- During the course of progestogen treatment endogenous FSH stimulates the initial growth and 'priming' of small follicles; LH concentrations in plasma are low.
- After termination of successful treatment, LH concentrations rise and cause follicular maturation and ovulation.

5.2 TO SHORTEN THE LUTEAL PHASE

This may be useful in a variety of circumstances including normal dioestrus, prolonged dioestrus and pregnancy up to 35 days (**17.2**, **20.3**).

- Prostaglandin (PG) (one dose is usually sufficient) causes prompt luteolysis and subsequent ovulation in 4–10 days, but the response may vary:
  (1) Prolonged dioestrus – if large follicles are present one may ovulate rapidly (24–48 hours after treatment) without the mare showing signs of heat, or she may be in oestrus for only 12–36 hours after ovulation.
  (2) Corpus haemorrhagicum/young corpus luteum (<6 days) will not respond to PG.
  (3) If the mare has had dioestrus ovulation (i.e. now has two CLs) the younger CL may not respond.
  (4) May cause sweating, transient diarrhoea and occasionally signs of colic.
- Mares with chronic obstructive pulmonary disease may exhibit respiratory embarrassment.
- Occasionally exogenous PG will not cause luteolysis; it is then necessary to dilate the cervix and irrigate the uterus with 250–500 ml warm saline. This may cause a transient vulval discharge.

5.3 TO HASTEN OVULATION

The optimal time for mating or insemination of a normal mare is 24–48 hours before ovulation. If ovulation could be hastened a more accurate breeding day might be predicted. In many cases these treatments are used as a 'holding injection', implying that they are given after breeding. The optimal use of these agents is part of a planned breeding regime.

Human chorionic gonadotrophin (hCG)

- Intravenous administration of hCG to oestrous mares with a follicle greater than 3.5 cm in diameter should result in ovulation within 48 hours.

- There is no guarantee that the mare will conceive; hCG only hastens ovulation and therefore reduces the requirement for repeated breedings.
- Anaphylactic reactions to hCG are rare.
- hCG antibodies are formed; these may theoretically reduce the effectiveness and/or compromise fertility; however, this has not been demonstrated to be a clinical problem.

Gonadotrophin releasing hormone (GnRH)

- GnRH is of limited value in inducing ovulation in mares.

Gonadotrophin releasing hormone agonists (buserelin, deslorelin)

- These agents may hasten ovulation in oestrous mares which have a preovulatory follicle greater than 3.5 cm in diameter.
- Buserelin is available for intravenous injection.
- Deslorelin is available (but not in the UK) as a subcutaneous implant.
- Antibody formation has not been demonstrated with these agents.

NB: The efficacy of any treatment designed to stimulate ovulation is difficult to assess as the drug is given at a time when ovulation would be expected anyway.

5.4 SYNCHRONISATION OF OVULATION

The oestrous cycle of the mare is characterised by a long and variable follicular phase. The time of ovulation is variable. Synchronisation of ovulation may be useful for batch artificial insemination or for embryo transfer.

A variety of methods are available, the commonest using progestogens.

- Progestogens must be administered for a prolonged period so that the only source of progesterone is the exogenous progestogen.
- One example is altrenogest for 14 days, prostaglandin on day 7 (to lyse any luteal tissue), and hCG on day 18. Ovulation would be expected on day 20, although this is not always the case.

6 The Optimum Time for Breeding and the Mating Procedure

6.1 THE OPTIMUM TIME FOR BREEDING

The mare ovulates secondary oocytes that are capable of being fertilised immediately. Oocytes retain maximal viability for only 12 hours after ovulation; however, it is clear that spermatozoa may survive for prolonged periods of time within the female reproductive tract. The optimum time for mating or insemination would therefore appear to be 24–48 hours before ovulation, this allowing time for spermatozoa to undergo capacitation. In the case of mares that have post-covering endometritis (see **13.2**, **15.2**) it may be appropriate for mating or insemination to occur earlier. A reduction in the pregnancy rate is, however, observed for matings that occur more than 4 days before ovulation.

A variation in the pregnancy rate to early matings is seen between stallions; spermatozoal longevity varies from one individual to another.

Matings that occur the day after ovulation are rarely fertile.

There are a number of techniques that may be used to identify the optimum time for mating. In many situations owners simply rely upon detection of oestrous behaviour; however, this may be unreliable. For optimum fertility there is no doubt that the prediction of ovulation using real-time diagnostic B-mode ultrasound imaging is the method of choice.

6.2 SIGNS OF OESTRUS

Mares vary in their willingness to show oestrus both from day to day, heat to heat and mare to mare. This may be influenced by teasing procedure.

- Some mares show readily to other mares and people, some show only to male horses and some will not show at all (**12.4**, **12.5**).
- Classical signs are: the mare straddles hind legs, raises tail, crouches slightly, urinates and persistently everts her clitoris (winking or showing).
- Some mares may 'wink' without urinating or lifting their tail.
- Other mares are simply less aggressive when teased.
- Mares rarely mount each other but occasionally mares in advanced pregnancy will mount mares in heat.

- Many shy or bad tempered mares 'show' better when twitched.
- Maiden mares often 'show' well but are difficult to cover without restraint.
- Some mares with foals 'show' best when the foal is present, others when it is out of earshot.
- Mares not in heat are either indifferent (especially in anoestrus) or violent, i.e. kick, bite, buck or strike out.

6.3 DETECTION OF OESTRUS

Oestrus may be detected by:

- seeing mare show spontaneously to an object, the owner or another horse
- a change of temperament – but this is often misleading, i.e. the owner thinks the mare is in heat when she is not
- a slight stickiness or yellow stain at the ventral commisure of the vulva
- some people who can smell a mare in heat
- clinical examination by a Veterinary Surgeon
- using a teaser, e.g.

  (1) the stallion by which the mare is to be covered
  (2) a teaser stallion kept for the purpose – cheaper to keep and easier to manage, especially if a pony is used
  (3) a gelding that is 'riggy'
  (4) a gelding that has been hormone (testosterone or oestrogen) treated, e.g. 200 mg testosterone subcutaneously
  (5) an unknown or unfamiliar mare or gelding.

6.4 TEASING TECHNIQUE

The object is to confront each mare individually with the teaser. The problem is that this is labour intensive and can be hazardous to personnel (foals also require restraint). The procedure usually requires 2–3 people.

- Ideally mares are teased at a board (teaser one side, mare the other) for at least 5 minutes. The initial reaction of the mare may be misleading.
- The teaser may be accommodated in a small enclosure, part of the side of which is a teasing board (with rail over to prevent teaser escaping). Mares are brought up to the board individually with the teaser unrestrained. The teaser may become difficult to handle.
- The teaser may be used in his own box in the same way, but the box door soon becomes damaged.
- The teaser, usually a pony, is walked through a field of mares and individuals are approached. There is some danger to the teaser and handler and teasing is not as thorough.

- Taking the teaser to fence or gate. Relies on mares approaching the teaser. Many mares will be 'missed' therefore this method is not recommended.
- Audio-tapes of stallion's calls may be played to mares, and their responses are observed.

6.5 DETECTION OF IMPENDING OVULATION

Impending ovulation may be predicted by manual and ultrasonographic examination of the reproductive tract performed *per rectum*.

- Follicles usually reach 4 cm in diameter before ovulating.
- Distinct softening of the follicle can be detected by palpation approximately 24 hours before ovulation.
- Follicle size can be accurately measured by using the electronic callipers of the ultrasound machine (remember the follicle has three dimensions).
- Follicle softening can be detected by ultrasound since the follicle appears to be flattened at the surface in contact with the ultrasound transducer (Fig. 6.1(a)).
- The follicle wall becomes increasingly echogenic prior to ovulation (Fig. 6.1(b)).
- Haemorrhage into the follicle occurs immediately prior to ovulation and this can be detected using ultrasound (Fig. 6.1(c)).
- A small outpouching of the follicle, directed towards the ovulation fossa, occurs as ovulation approaches (Fig. 6.1(d)).
- The uterus of the mare becomes oedematous during oestrus. This oedema can be detected and the amount of oedema can be characterised using ultrasound (Fig. 6.2). In the majority of mares the degree of oedema reduces 24 hours before ovulation.

The clinical and ultrasound features should be used in combination with each other rather than in isolation.

On stud farms in which regular examination of mares is performed it is possible to abolish completely the requirement for routine teasing of mares (other than immediately prior to covering).

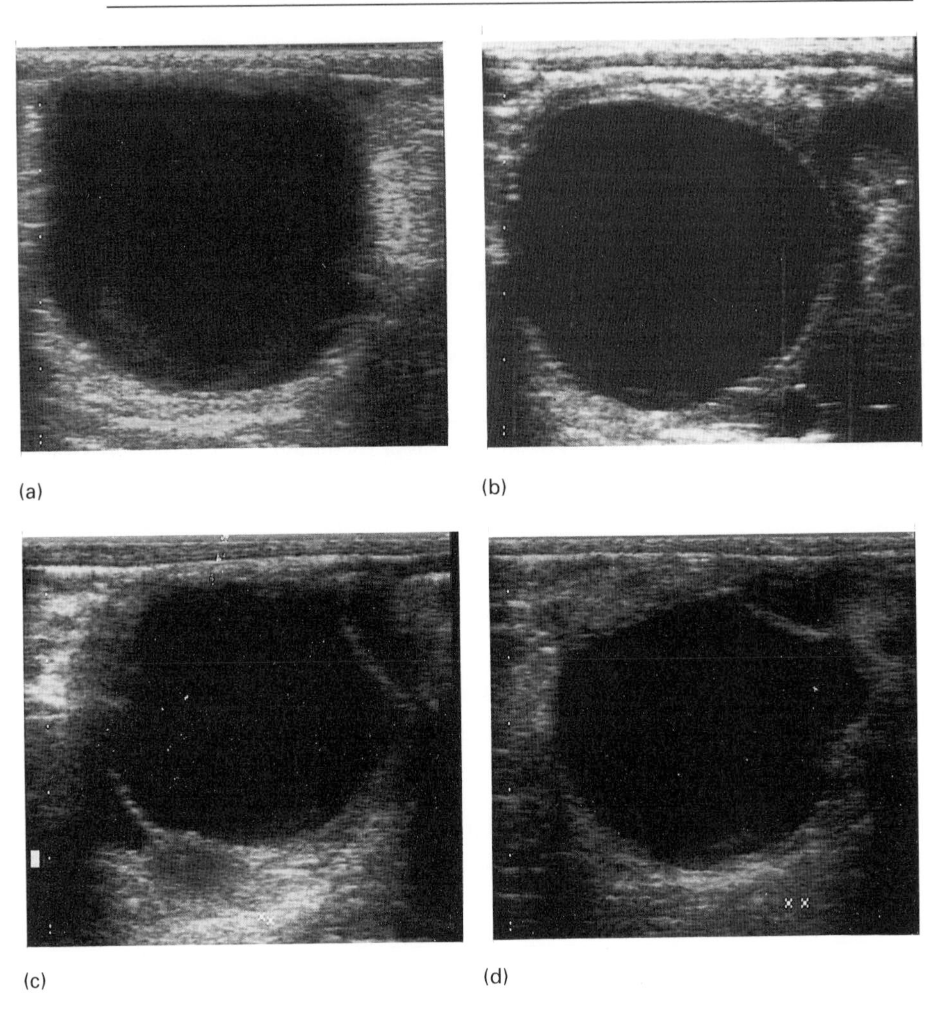

Fig. 6.1. Ultrasound images of follicles prior to ovulation demonstrating signs that may be useful for the prediction of the time of ovulation (7.5 MHz transducer, scale in cm). (a) Flattening of the follicle (indicative of follicular softening); (b) increased echogenicity of the follicular wall; (c) presence of haemorrhage (small echogenic particles) within the follicular fluid; (d) outpouching of the follicle directed towards the ovulation fossa.

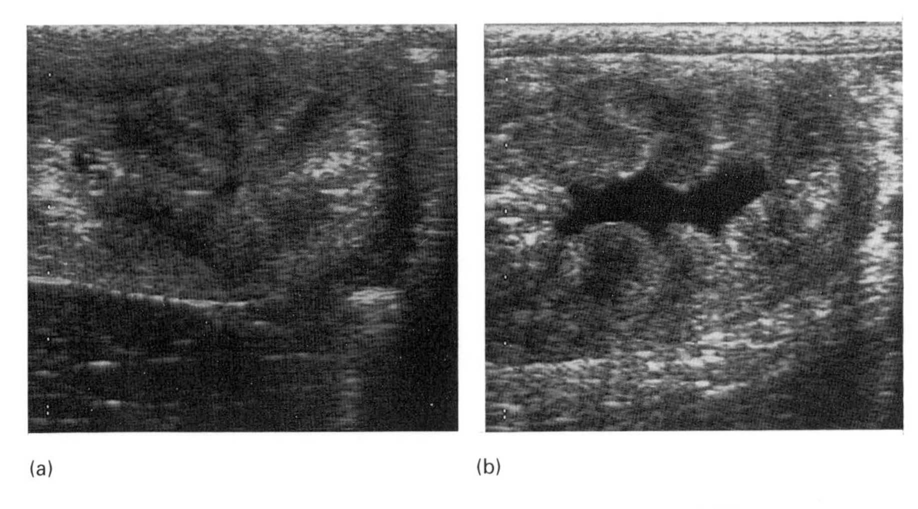

(a) (b)

Fig. 6.2. Ultrasound images of the uterus during oestrus (7.5 MHz transducer, scale in cm); (a) Slight amount of oedema within the endometrium; (b) marked endometrial oedema. In general, mares reach a peak of uterine oedema which declines 24 hours before ovulation.

6.6 RESTRAINT OF THE MARE FOR MATING

Ideally this should be minimal but since the stallion is usually more valuable and vulnerable than the mare, some restraint is usually used.

- For a quiet mare, known to be 'well in season', a head collar or bridle is sufficient.
- A twitch is usually sufficient for a slightly nervous mare, or one 'going off'. It is essential for a mare of unknown temperament. It is easier if the mare is to stand in a preselected position, e.g. in a hollow to allow mating by a smaller stallion. Use a twitch with a short handle which clips onto the head collar, or a very long handle so that holder can stand well clear of fore-limbs.
- Felt or canvas/leather boots help take the force out of the kick. They are slightly hazardous to apply and remove. The mare often 'dances' due to unfamiliar sensation and may kick until they come off. They often come off if the mare moves frequently.
- Hobbles with side lines almost completely prevent the mare from kicking (Fig. 6.3) but:

  (1) they are hazardous to apply to a difficult mare;
  (2) they must have a quick release mechanism on the mare's chest in case mare and/or stallion become entangled.

- Lifting the left fore-leg with a rope or special leather leg strap with quick release mechanism – release when stallion has mounted or if the mare stumbles. This method is useful for a maiden mare that tries to run forward or buck.

- Low doses of the α_2-adrenoceptor agonists (detomidine, romifidine, xylazine) may be useful as these are anxiolytic. The mare may become too ataxic if high doses are used.
- Stallions' instinct. Some stallions take measures to avoid being kicked by:

  (1) mounting the mare from side or quarters and then swivelling round to the right position – stallion may get both feet over the mare's back and be forced to dismount
  (2) biting the mare's lower left leg just before mounting – she lifts the leg and is off balance
  (3) nudging the mare's left hip with right shoulder just before mounting – the mare is off balance.

- Bandaging the mare's tail helps to prevent hairs from being introduced into the vulva and allows the stallion handler to observe the position of the horse's penis.
  NB: Do not clean the mare's vulva with antiseptic. If necessary remove gross contamination with water and dry well.

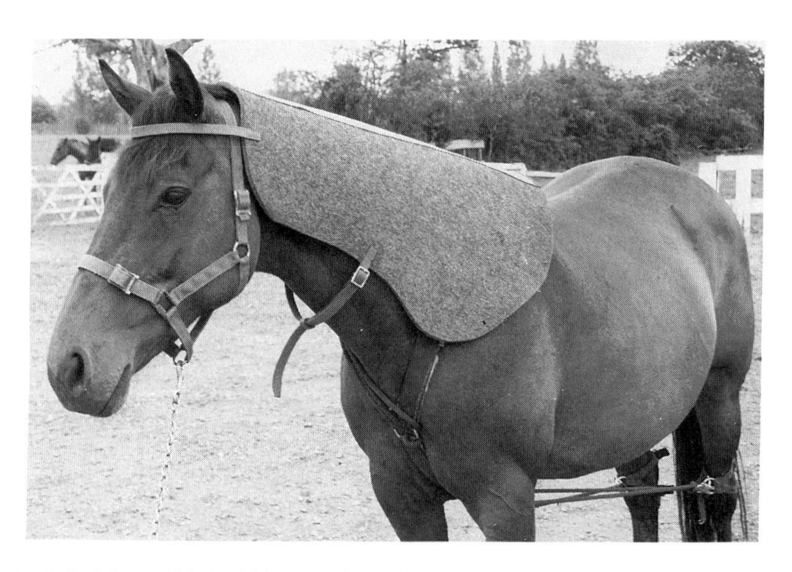

Fig. 6.3. Mare with hobbles and a collar.

6.7 INJURIES DURING MATING

Stallion

Usually traumatic due to:

(1) kicks on the penis or back leg (stifle joint)
(2) haematoma in the corpus cavernosum of the penis due to the mare twisting sideways suddenly during mating
(3) stallion slipping and falling.

- Any injury to the penis usually causes prolapse and swelling (haematoma and oedema). Treatment is conservative, i.e. cold water, support for the penis and protection from excoriation. Do not give tranquillisers.
- Inguinal or scrotal hernia can occur during mating.
- Laceration to the dorsum of the penis due to sutures in the mare's vulva.
- Psychological damage, particularly to young horses, due to a rough handler or mare.
- Fatal haemorrhage, due to rupture of the aorta, occurs rarely.

Mare

The mare may be either bitten, or damaged by the stallion's penis.

Bites

- Most stallions nip the mare's buttocks, flanks and legs before mounting. Some stallions bite the mare's neck during mating.
- Bites at the rear end rarely cause trouble but occasionally a stallion appears to dislike a mare, and bites her savagely without mounting.
- Stallion may cause obvious trauma to the mare's neck; this is avoided by:

  (1) placing a stick between the stallion's teeth when he tries to bite
  (2) covering the mare's neck with a sack, cloth or a leather collar.

Vaginal trauma

Clinical signs are haemorrhage and straining due to:

(1) rupture of hymen remnants in maidens (**12.15**)
(2) rupture of vagina – usually dorsal or lateral fornix and retro-peritoneal. If rupture is diagnosed, give parenteral antibiotics
(3) cervical damage and rupture of the uterus; these are rare.

- Some stallions commonly cause vaginal trauma due to either large penis or dorsal thrusting.
- Trauma can be avoided by inserting a padded cylinder (breeder's roll) between the stallion's abdomen and the mare's rump during coitus; this reduces the length of the penis in the vagina.

6.8 PSYCHOLOGICAL PROBLEMS AT MATING

- Some stallions may find certain mares 'unattractive' and be disinclined to mate with them.
- Excessive checking of the stallion may cause loss of erection and disinclination to mount.
- Drenching the mare's hindquarters in urine from another mare in heat may induce the stallion to cover the mare normally.

7 Normal Pregnancy

7.1 ANATOMICAL AND MORPHOLOGICAL CHANGES OF THE UTERUS

There are characteristic changes of the reproductive tract that occur during pregnancy.

- The uterus becomes progressively more turgid, tubular (tonic) and more narrow from about 15 days to 21 days post-ovulation.
- By 21 days the uterine body and horns feel sausage or hose-pipe like due to increased tone. These changes are not specific for pregnancy however:

  (1) tone may not be marked in older parous mares or maiden mares
  (2) post-partum involution may produce turgidity similar to the tone of pregnancy
  (3) acute endometritis causes turgidity similar to pregnancy
  (4) the uterus is tonic in some cases of prolonged dioestrus.

- At about 21 days the conceptual swelling develops at the base of one of the uterine horns. This swelling is 3 to 5 cm in diameter and it bulges ventrally.
- The uterine wall over the conceptus is thin, but the persistent tone in the adjacent uterus keeps the conceptus in place after day 16 (Fig. 7.1).
- As the conceptus grows the swelling becomes larger but remains roughly spherical. The distal part of the pregnant horn remains tonic.
- By 60 days the swelling is about 12 cm in diameter and fills the pregnant horn. The body and non-pregnant horn are still tonic.
- After 60 days the swelling usually becomes less tense and starts to involve the body and eventually the non-pregnant horn.
- By 90 days the whole uterus is filled with fluid (**8.2**).
- Further distension of the uterus causes the ventral surface of the uterine body to lie against the ventral body wall. The dorsal surface of the uterus is suspended by the broad ligaments.
- Distinction between body and horns becomes less obvious.
- At day 36 endometrial cups start to develop in a ring round the equator of the conceptus.

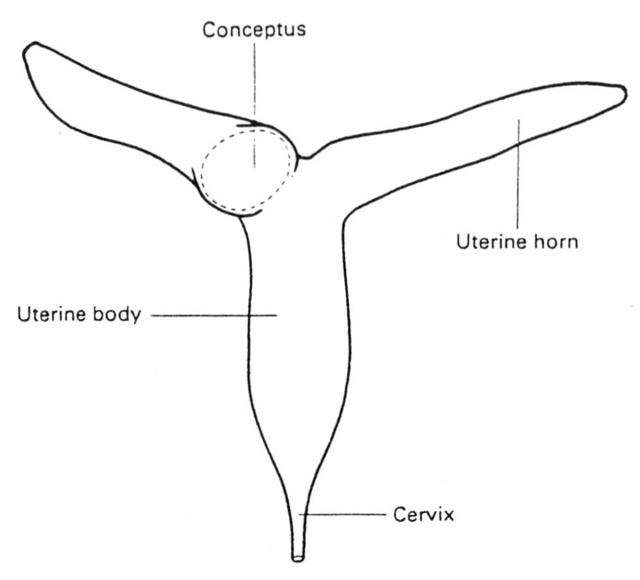

Fig. 7.1. The conceptus becomes fixed at the base of one of the uterine horns on the 16th day after ovulation.

- The endometrial cups produce equine chorionic gonadotrophin (eCG) (previously termed pregnant mare serum gonadotrophin (PMSG)).
- As the conceptus becomes larger, cups are adjacent to its dorsal aspect. NB: cups are not palpable *per rectum*.
- At 100–150 days the cups become necrotic and slough off the surface of the endometrium, and come to lie between that and the allantochorion.
- Invaginations develop in the allantochorion to accommodate the dead cup tissue – these become chorio-allantoic pouches or vesicles (Fig. 7.2).

7.2 DEVELOPMENT OF THE CONCEPTUS

- Sufficient spermatozoa for fertilisation are present within the uterine (Fallopian) tubes by 4–6 hours after coitus.
- The ovum is fertilised in the uterine tube to produce the conceptus.
- The conceptus reaches the uterus about 5–6 days after ovulation.
- Non-fertilised ova remain in the uterine tube and degenerate.
- The conceptus is mobile in the uterine horns and body for up to 16 days.
- The conceptus at this early stage is principally a yolk sac filled bag.
- The mobility phase is important for the maternal recognition of pregnancy.
- The conceptus then becomes lodged at the base of one of the uterine horns, usually the narrower one (not related to the side of ovulation).

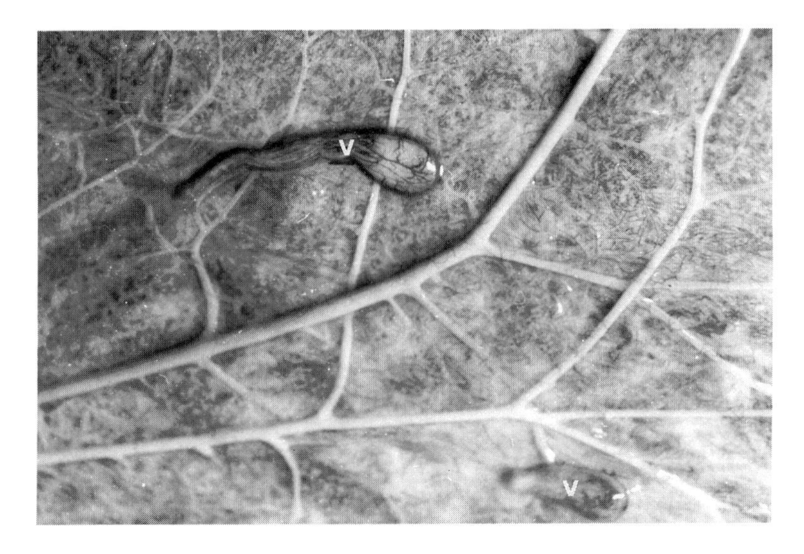

Fig. 7.2. Chorio-allantoic vesicles (v) on the inner surface of the allantochorion.

- The embryo develops on the ventral aspect of the conceptus and is free of the trophoblast wall by 20 days.
- Development of early allantois between the embryo and trophoblast raises the embryo dorsally (Fig. 7.3).
- As the yolk sac (which is dorsal to the embryo) becomes smaller and the allantois becomes larger, the embryo moves further dorsally within the conceptus.
- The mesoderm surrounding the yolk sac carries blood vessels.
- The umbilicus will be attached dorsally (at the base of one uterine horn).
- After about 35 days, most organogenesis is completed and the embryo is called a fetus.
- The fetus remains in the uterine horn until about 70–80 days, but is then usually in the body until 6–7 months.
- By now the fetus is becoming too large to remain only in the body, and its hind quarters begin to occupy one horn, usually the original pregnant horn.
- After this time the fetus cannot change its presentation.
- Until just before the second stage of parturition, the fetus usually lies in a ventral or lateral position with limbs, head and neck flexed.

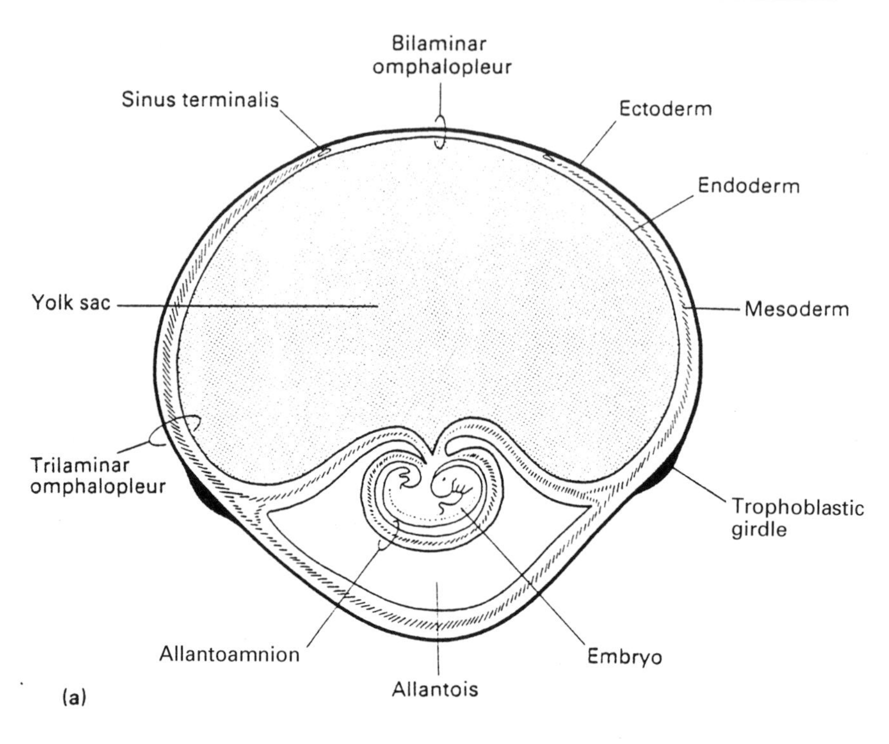
Bilaminar
omphalopleur
Sinus terminalis
Ectoderm
Endoderm
Yolk sac
Mesoderm
Trilaminar
omphalopleur
Trophoblastic
girdle
Allantoamnion
Embryo
Allantois
(a)

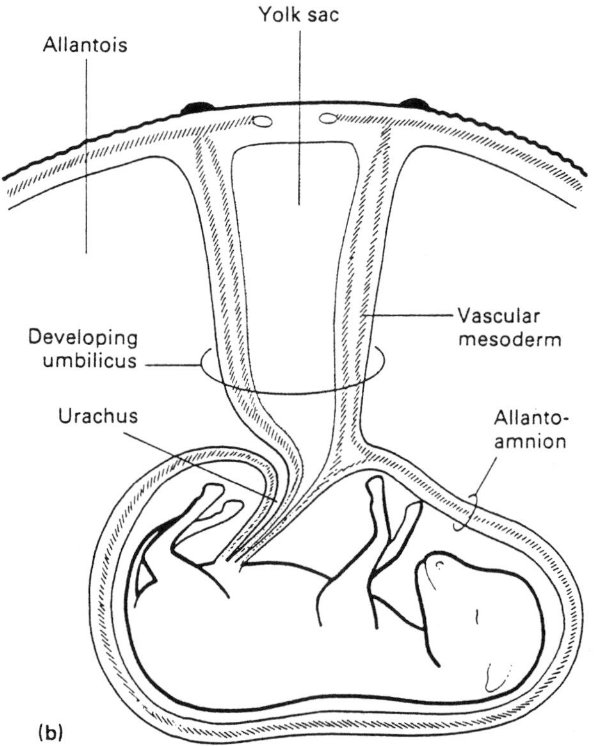
Yolk sac
Allantois
Vascular
mesoderm
Developing
umbilicus
Urachus
Allanto-
amnion
(b)

7.3 PLACENTA AND FETAL MEMBRANES

Placenta

The placenta of the mare is epitheliochorial (no loss of maternal tissue) and diffuse (throughout the whole uterus, except at the cervix and the uterine ends of the uterine tube).

- Villi of trophoblast from the chorion occupy crypts in microcotyledons of the endometrium; the placenta is described as being microcotyledonary.
- Placental attachment begins around 25 days and becomes more extensive as the allantochorion fills more of the uterine lumen.
- Physical attachment of the placenta is not strong, as diffuse placentation allows adequate surface area for physiological function.
- Physical stability of the placenta is aided by:

  (1) tone of uterus adjacent to the conceptus in the early stages
  (2) large volume of fluid keeping whole of the uterus distended in later stages.

- Weak physical attachment of the placenta ensures easy separation of the allantochorion from the endometrium in the third stage of parturition (**9.6**).

Fetal membranes

Fetal membranes consist of:

- The *allantochorion* or *chorio-allantoic membrane* (CAM). The outer surface of this membrane (chorion) is covered with micro-villi which are composed of capillaries, a little stromal tissue, and an epithelium. This surface looks velvet-like and is red in colour. The inner surface is shiny, and through it can be seen the larger veins and arteries which emanate from the umbilical vessels.
- The *amnion*, which is formed by fusion of the allantois and amnion proper (this membrane would more correctly be called the allanto-amnion). It is an opaque white membrane containing many tortuous blood vessels (these become straighter as pregnancy progresses)
- The amnion and CAM are completely separate from each other, and are only attached indirectly via the umbilical cord.
- The umbilical cord traverses the allantoic cavity, and at the level of the amnion, the two veins join to form one vessel in the amniotic cavity.

Fig. 7.3. (a) Diagram of an equine conceptus at 30 days; the developing allantois is pushing the embryo dorsally and the vascular mesoderm is enveloping the yolk sac. (b) Diagram of part of the equine conceptus at 55 days; the yolk sac is becoming vestigial and will be enveloped by the blood vessels of the umbilical cord.

- The amniotic part of the cord also contains the urachus, a canal which conducts fetal urine from the bladder to the allantoic cavity.
- The amniotic cord, and inner surface of the amnion, are often covered with small rough plaques of cells which contain glycogen.
- Twisting of the umbilical cord and/or dilations of the urachus are often associated with abortion (**18.5**).
- The *hippomanes* is a soft calculus of cellular and inorganic debris which forms in the allantoic cavity. Occasionally there are accessory small hippomanes either free in the fluid or attached to the CAM particularly on the chorio-allantoic pouches (wrongly called 'false hippomanes').

7.4 ENDOCRINOLOGY OF PREGNANCY

The major hormonal events during gestation are as follows.

Progesterone

Concentrations (from the primary corpus luteum or CL verum) usually fall slightly at 14–16 days post-ovulation, but are rarely less than 1 ng/ml plasma. They may also fall again around the 30th–40th day. Thereafter values rise due to:

- stimulation of greater progesterone output from the primary CL by eCG (PMSG)
- both ovulation and luteinisation of follicles forming secondary progesterone producing CLs and luteinised follicles.

Progesterone thereafter is also produced by the placenta (both fetal and maternal components), so that when the CLs regress from about 120 days, pregnancy is maintained by placental progesterone.

- Placental progesterone acts locally, so blood concentrations are low after 5 months.
- Progesterone concentrations in blood rise just before parturition.

Luteinising hormone

LH concentrations are low throughout gestation.

Follicle stimulating hormone

FSH is released episodically up to 40 days and probably also to about 100 days.

- Before 40 days it is responsible for follicular development, and thereafter is probably synergistic with eCG in causing marked ovarian activity.

Oestrogen

There are several sources of oestrogen in the pregnant mare.

1. Oestrogens produced by the early conceptus. Oestrogen producing capability occurs as early as day 12. These oestrogens are locally produced and do not increase circulating concentrations.
2. Oestrogens produced by the ovary. These increase at approximately the time that eCG is produced from the endometrial cups.
3. Oestrogens produced by the feto-placental unit. These increase after day 60. The large amount of oestrogen in late pregnancy is produced by the fetal gonads.

In general until approximately day 80 plasma oestrogen concentrations are low; thereafter vast quantities of equilin, equilenin, oestrone and 17-β oestradiol may be detected.

- Both blood and urine concentrations of these oestrogens remain high until 300 days, after which they decline to parturition.
- Oestrone is conjugated to oestrone sulphate in the fetal liver; the amount of this hormone in the maternal circulation is an indication of fetal 'wellbeing'.

Equine chorionic gonadotrophin (eCG) or PMSG

This is produced by the endometrial cups and appears in the circulation at about day 40. Values rise rapidly to peak at 60–70 days and thereafter decline.

- There is marked individual variation in the amount and length of time for which eCG is produced, e.g. it may disappear by 80 days or still be present at 150 days.

7.5 CERVICAL CHANGES

- In early pregnancy the cervix appears identical to dioestrus (**4.6**) but at speculum examination may be deflected up, down or laterally. This is because the cervix is stuck to the vaginal wall by mucus.
- As pregnancy progresses, the anterior vagina and external os of the cervix become covered in very tacky, dry mucus.
- After the fifth month the cervix becomes softer and shorter possibly due to high concentrations of circulating oestrogens.
- NB: A finger can be passed along the cervical canal at all stages of pregnancy. This is undesirable as pregnancy failure follows due to introduction of infection or (in later pregnancy) rupture of the allanto-chorion.

7.6 OVARIAN CHANGES

- Primary corpus luteum (CL) of pregnancy (*corpus luteum verum*) is not lysed at 14 days and persist until 120–150 days.

- 18–40 days: ovaries are characterised by the presence of many (up to 3 cm diameter) follicles. Ovulations are uncommon.
- 40–120 days: extensive ovarian activity with multi-follicular development, ovulations and luteinisation of unruptured follicles. Secondary corpora lutea are formed.
- 120 days to term: follicular activity ceases, all corpora lutea regress and ovaries become small and inactive.
- The position of ovaries up to 2 months of pregnancy is as for the non-pregnant mare. Thereafter they are pulled cranially and medially but remain dorsal to the uterus. Tension on the utero-ovarian ligaments makes the ovaries less mobile. The ovaries are not usually palpable after 5 months because they are difficult to reach.

7.7 MULTIPLE CONCEPTUSES (COMMONLY TWINS) (18.4, 20.2)

- Twin pregnancy is undesirable in the mare as it often terminates in the abortion of both fetuses, or the birth of dead fetuses, or undernourished live foals at term.
- Equine twins are dizygotic, i.e. from two ova. Commonly they originate from separate follicles; therefore multiple corpora lutea are present. In less than 50% of cases they develop one in each horn, in the others two conceptuses are adjacent to each other at the base of the same horn.
- In some cases early death of one embryo and subsequent resorption allows the other conceptus to develop normally.
- Conceptuses that both develop past 60 days compete for placental space, resulting in:

  (1) early death of one small conceptus trapped at the tip of the uterine horn. May be evidence of this when the other (normal) foal is born at term (do not mistake these for fetal 'moles' which are yolk sac anomalies, not twins)
  (2) death of one fetus later, followed by continuation of the pregnancy and the production of an undernourished live foal near or after term with a fetal 'mummy'
  (3) death of one fetus later, followed by abortion of both fetuses, one usually alive. This occurs when the viable pregnancy is unable to produce enough progesterone to maintain pregnancy.

- Diagnosis of twin pregnancy (**20.2**).
- Management of twin pregnancy (**20.1**, **20.3**).
- NB: udder development and milk production during gestation often denotes (a) death of a twin and may be followed by abortion or survival of the other fetus, (b) placental separation due to other causes.

7.8 DURATION OF PREGNANCY

- Pregnancy length is of the order of 330–345 days in the mare, but is very variable, with extremes of 310–370 days or even longer occurring not infrequently.
- Factors which affect pregnancy length are:

  (1) date of conception; mares which conceive (and therefore foal) early in the year have longer gestation lengths, probably because maximum growth of the foal occurs when natural food (grass) is not available and nutrition may be poor
  (2) sex of foal; male foals have gestation lengths about 1 day longer than females on average
  (3) individual variation; some mares have similar gestation lengths (e.g. consistently over 12 months) in successive pregnancies, but others do not
  (4) placental lesions may cause retardation of the growth of the fetus and an extension in pregnancy length. The foal may still be dysmature at birth
  (5) death of one twin and continuation of pregnancy may result in growth retardation of the fetus.

- Problems associated with pregnancies which exceed expected duration are (**9.3**):

  (1) mainly owner orientated, e.g. owner sat up or took time off work, etc. for expected foaling which did not occur
  (2) foal may be oversized and cause dystocia – this is rare. Most long pregnancies are essential to ensure that the foal is mature at birth, and dysmature foals may be produced after a normal length of pregnancy, or even after an extended pregnancy
  (3) foal may be dead and mummifying or putrifying, etc. Unfounded fear as death of a single fetus invariably results in rapid abortion (**17.3**, **17.4**).

- NB: mares will foal when they are ready, not necessarily when they are calculated to be 'due'.

8 Pregnancy Diagnosis

Pregnancy diagnosis is necessary for management and husbandry reasons. The early diagnosis of pregnancy is particularly important if the method of diagnosis can distinguish between single and multiple conceptuses. Later pregnancy diagnosis is also important since early embryonic death is not uncommon in the mare, and the development of pseudopregnancy may compromise the fertility of a mare in a given breeding season.

8.1 ABSENCE OF SUBSEQUENT OESTRUS

This method is commonly (unwittingly) used by stud personnel and owners as an initial screening method. However:

- Some mares show oestrous behaviour when pregnant, and these mares may be mated especially if restrained: this may cause embryonic death, if the cervix is opened during coitus – more likely in old or recently foaled mares.
- It is commonly assumed that the mare will be in oestrus 21 days after mating and this is not necessarily true (**2.2**). Teasing may therefore be too late in either normal or short cycles.
- If the mare returns home after mating the owners may not be able to recognise oestrus. This is especially true when there is no stallion or other appropriate stimulus.
- Some mares which return to oestrus after mating may show no signs, especially those with foals (silent heat – **12.4**).
- Non-pregnant mares may not return to heat, usually due to prolonged dioestrus (**4.9**) and occasionally due to anoestrus (at the end of the season or during periods of inclement weather).
- Non-pregnant mares may occasionally enter lactational anoestrus especially if foaling in January–March.
- Non-pregnant mares may not demonstrate oestrous behaviour if they are protective of their foal.

8.2 CLINICAL EXAMINATION

- Ovarian palpation contributes little to pregnancy diagnosis as large follicles may be (and often are) present, and the CL is not palpable.
- Uterine and cervical changes are described in **7.1** and **7.5**.
- At 18–21 days: good uterine tone and a tightly closed cervix (as assessed *per rectum* or *vaginam*) are indicators of pregnancy.
- 21–60 days: good uterine tone, swelling at the base of one or both (twins) uterine horns and tightly closed cervix. All must be present for positive diagnosis.
- 60–120 days: swelling becomes less discrete, uterine horns become more difficult to palpate and uterine body becomes more fluid filled and prominent. May be intrapelvic and tense in young mares. This is often a difficult time for pregnancy diagnosis. Continuity with the cervix helps identification of the uterus. Fetus can sometimes be balloted (**7.1**, **7.2**).
- 120 days to term: cervix becomes softer, fetus becomes more obvious. Dorsal surface of uterine body always in reach. Fetus often felt moving after 6 months.
- *Optimum time for rectal examination* depends on:

  (1) experience of clinician – later examinations (40 to 60 days) are usually easiest
  (2) time of year – the later the examination the more time is lost if the mare is not pregnant.
  (3) value of mare – early positive examinations should be repeated to detect pregnancy failure. Repeat examinations are recommended up to 40 days. After this pregnancy failure is rarely followed by a fertile oestrus (**17.5**).

8.3 PROGESTERONE CONCENTRATIONS

Progesterone concentrations in plasma (or milk) can be measured by:

1. *Radio-immunoassay:* sample must be sent (delivered) to laboratory and the result may take two or more days to obtain.
2. *Enzyme-linked immunosorbent assay (ELISA) tests:* these can be conducted in a practice laboratory and the results are rapidly obtained (horse plasma can be harvested in 30 minutes without a centrifuge). The cost per sample is lowest when many samples are assayed in a batch (standards do not need repeating).

- At 18–20 days post-ovulation pregnant mares should have plasma progesterone concentration above 1 ng/ml
  BUT
- not all mares with high progesterone are pregnant (cf. prolonged dioestrus, early fetal death and mares with short cycles)

- mis-timing of sampling (relative to previous ovulation) will give erroneous results
- occasionally pregnant mares have low progesterone concentrations for short periods of time
- thorough clinical examination gives cheaper and more complete and accurate information on the mare's reproductive status.

8.4 EQUINE CHORIONIC GONADOTROPHIN

Equine chorionic gonadotrophin (eCG, PMSG) appears in the blood in detectable concentrations at approximately 40 days after ovulation and usually persists until 80–120 days after ovulation. The hormone is produced by the endometrial cups (**7.4**).

The amount of eCG produced varies greatly from mare to mare, and mares carrying multiple conceptuses do not necessarily produce more than those with singleton pregnancies.

- Errors in the test are due to:

  (1) sampling at the wrong time
  (2) some mares producing little eCG after 80 days
  (3) mares in which pregnancy fails after the endometrial cups form continuing to produce eCG (false positive) (**17.5**)
  (4) possible loss of potency in samples not tested immediately.

- eCG can be detected by radio-immunoassay (commercial laboratories), haemagglutination-inhibition test (commercial laboratories and test kit for practitioners), and latex agglutination test (test kit for practitioners).

8.5 PLACENTAL OESTROGENS

These reach peak levels in plasma and urine at 150 days, and concentrations remain high until after 300 days. The amount of oestrogen produced is so great that false positives do not occur due to other conditions. False negative results are also very rare after 150 days. Oestrogens are tested for in the urine – free oestrogens produce a colour reaction with sulphuric acid. The Cuboni test is the most accurate but involves an extraction procedure using benzene (carcinogen) and acid. The Lunaas test is simpler, uses acids but is sometimes difficult to interpret.

Plasma. Assays for oestrone sulphate are now commercially available.

8.6 ULTRASOUND EXAMINATION

The early diagnosis of pregnancy with ultrasound is highly accurate although there are several potential pitfalls including the confusion of uterine cysts for conceptuses and the presence of multiple conceptuses.

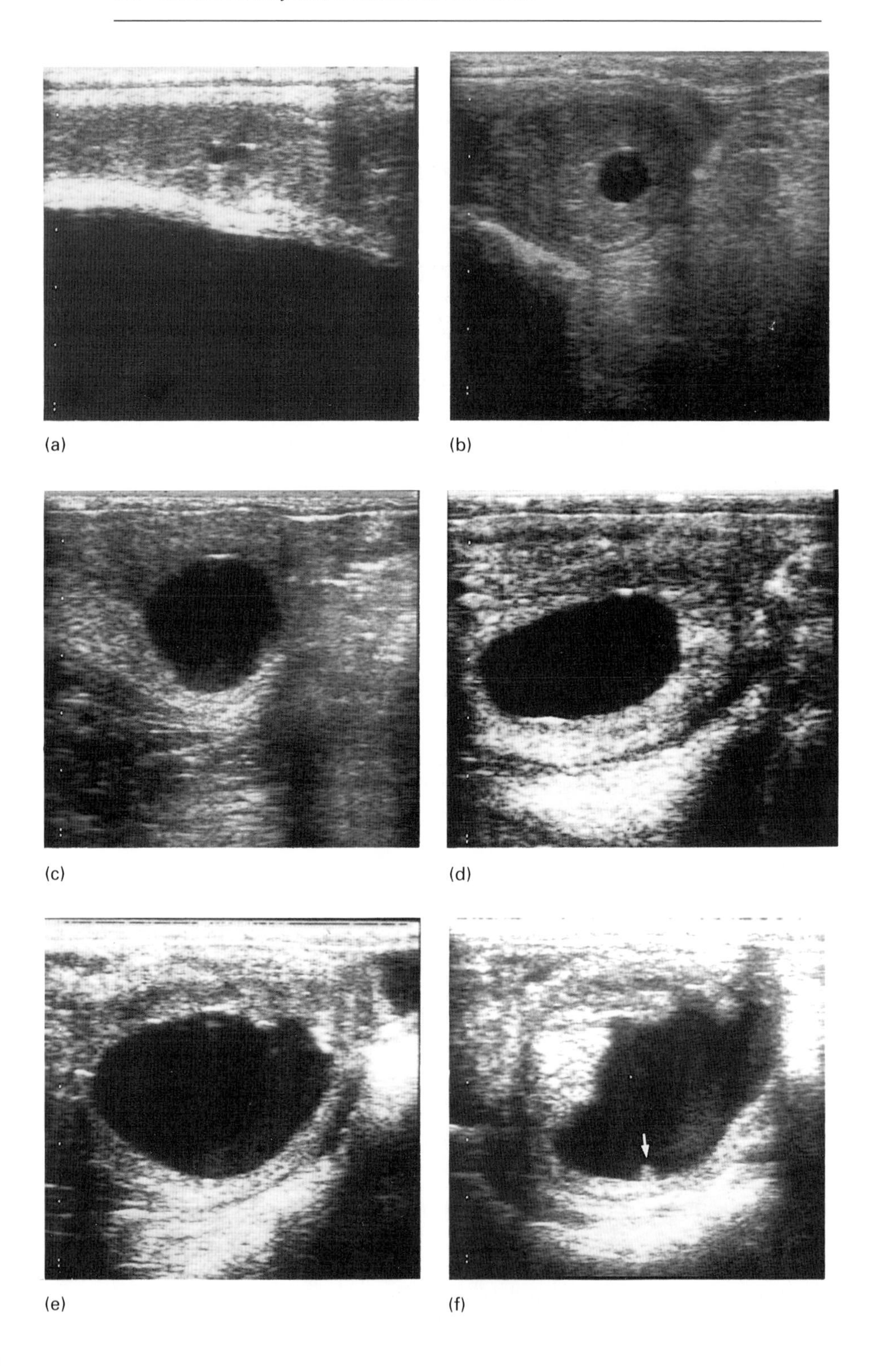
(a)
(b)
(c)
(d)
(e)
(f)

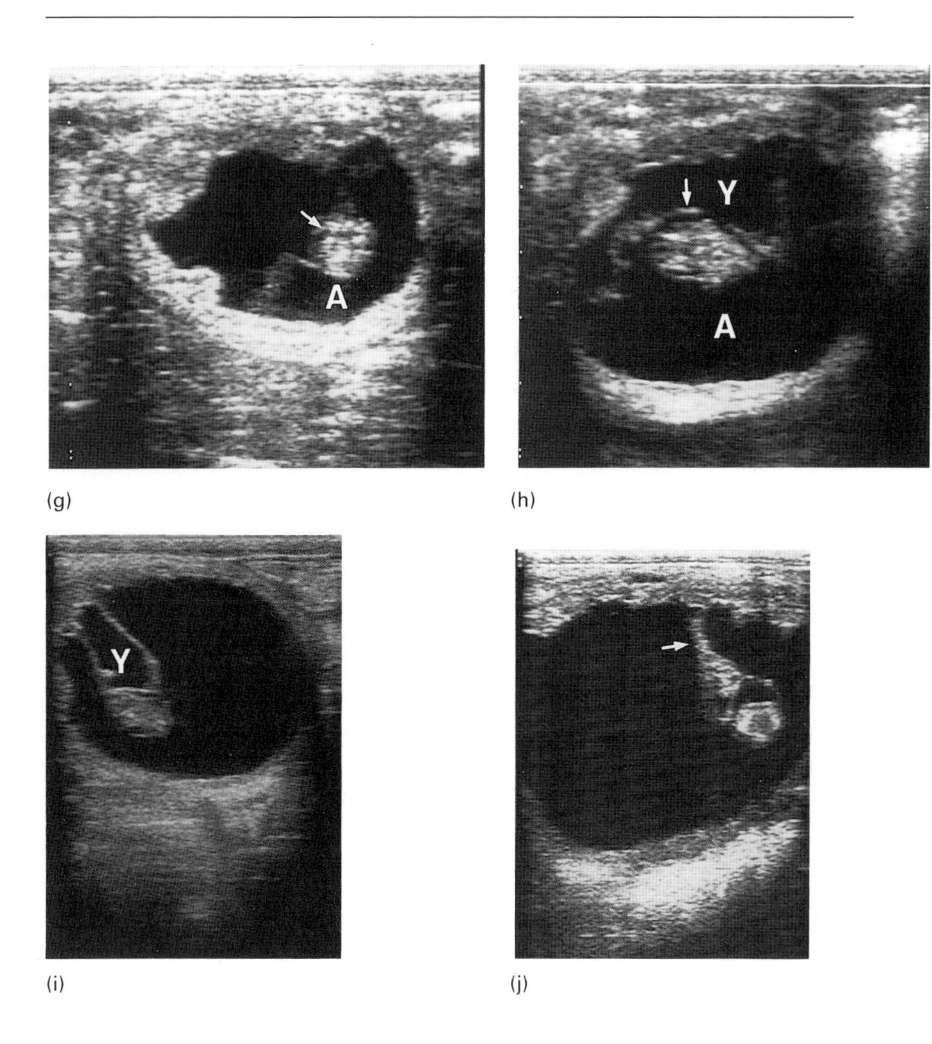

Fig. 8.1. Ultrasound images of equine pregnancy (7.5 MHz transducer, scale in cm).
(a) Anechoic conceptus 12 days after ovulation (present in the body of the uterus). (b) Conceptus at 14 days after ovulation (present in the tip of one uterine horn). (c) Conceptus at 16 days after ovulation. (d) Conceptus at 18 days after ovulation: the conceptus is no longer spherical. (e) Conceptus at 20 days after ovulation. (f) Conceptus at 21 days after ovulation: the embryo is visible on the ventral pole of the conceptus (arrow), protruding into the yolk sac. (g) Conceptus 25 days after ovulation: the allantois (A) has increased in volume and the embryo has been pushed dorsally (arrow); the volume of the yolk sac is decreasing. (h) Conceptus at 32 days after ovulation: the allantois (A) is larger in volume than the yolk sac (Y), the amnion (arrow) can now be imaged. (i) Conceptus at 35 days after ovulation: the yolk sac (Y) has almost been obliterated. Note the change in scale compared with previous images. (j) Conceptus at 40 days after ovulation: the forming umbilicus is visible (arrow).

Diagnosis of early pregnancy (Fig. 8.1)

The early conceptus can be imaged when there is sufficient yolk sac fluid to be imaged. The yolk sac appears as an anechoic structure which in early pregnancy is spherical. There is usually a small echogenic region on the dorsal and ventral pole of the conceptus; this is a normal ultrasound artifact.

- From 10 days after ovulation the conceptus can be imaged; it appears as a spherical anechoic structure approximately 2 mm in diameter.
- The conceptus rapidly increases in diameter to reach approximately 10 mm in diameter 14 days after ovulation. The outline remains circular (spherical) presumably because of the thick embryonic capsule.
- Until day 16 the conceptus is mobile and may be identified either within the uterine horns or the uterine body. This mobile phase is important for the maternal recognition of pregnancy.
- During pregnancy diagnosis careful attention to imaging of the entire uterus is required; the transducer should be moved slowly from the tip of one uterine horn to the other, and then caudally towards the cervix.
- Trans-uterine migration usually ceases by day 17, and the conceptus becomes fixed in position at the base of one uterine horn.
- From day 17 until day 28 the increase in conceptus diameter is slowed.
- After fixation the conceptus rotates so that its thickest portion, the region of the embryonic pole, assumes a ventral position.
- The uterine wall adjacent to the dorsal pole of the conceptus becomes thickened.
- The conceptus generally retains a spherical outline until approximately 17 days after ovulation after which time it may be deformed by pressure from the transducer; it may then appear triangular or flattened in outline.
- The embryo may be imaged from approximately 21 days after ovulation when it appears as an oblong shaped hyperechoic structure adjacent to the ventral pole of the conceptus.
- A heart beat is commonly detected within the embryonic mass from approximately 22 days after ovulation. This structure appears as a rapidly flickering motion in the central portion of the embryonic mass.
- Growth of the allantois lifts the embryo from the ventral position and the allantois *per se* may be identified from day 24, when it appears as an anechoic structure ventral to the embryo (**7.2**).
- The size of the allantois increases and that of the yolk sac is gradually reduced until at approximately 30 days after ovulation they are similar in volume.
- From day 30 onwards it is possible to image the amnion surrounding the developing embryo.
- At 35 days after ovulation the embryo is approximately 15 mm in length and the allantois is three times the volume of the yolk sac.

- By days 38–40 the fetus is positioned adjacent to the dorsal pole of the conceptus.
- At day 40 the yolk sac is almost completely absent, and the umbilicus which attaches to the dorsal pole can be imaged.

Diagnosis of pregnancy from day 40 after ovulation (Fig. 8.2)

Imaging of the pregnancy after the formation of the endometrial cups may be necessary to ensure continued fetal development and to assess fetal viability. This may be of value when there is concern of fetal resorption or abortion or when multiple conceptuses have been managed.

- Pregnancy diagnosis with ultrasound at this stage is highly accurate.
- Later however it may be difficult to appreciate fully the presence of multiple conceptuses.
- From day 40 after ovulation the yolk sac is collapsed and almost completely obliterated. The umbilicus which incorporates the yolk sac is tortuous and appears relatively hyperechoic.
- The umbilicus remains attached to the dorsal pole of the conceptus; it increases in length allowing the fetus to move to a ventral position within the conceptus.
- The fetus is positioned adjacent to the ventral pole from 50 days after ovulation.
- After day 50 limb buds can be readily imaged and ballottement of the uterus causes the fetus to float within the allantoic fluid; fetal movements are commonly seen.
- The abdominal and thoracic portions of the fetus can be differentiated after day 50.
- Imaging of the fetal stomach is possible after day 60. The stomach is variably filled with anechoic fluid and can be detected caudal to the liver in more than 90% of fetuses.
- The fetal eyes may be imaged from day 60 and measurement of their diameter may be used to estimate the gestational age.

Diagnosis of late pregnancy (Fig. 8.3)

Late examinations using ultrasound may not be necessary since pregnancy diagnosis is simple by palpation at this time. However, ultrasound is being used increasingly to confirm normal fetal development, and to assess fetal wellbeing.

- The fetal skeleton becomes visible during late pregnancy; the head, spinal column and ribs produce intense reflections that are easily identifiable.
- From 150 days onwards it is not always possible to image the entire fetus using high frequency transducers because of their short depth of penetration. The dorsal portion of the fluid filled uterus can always be

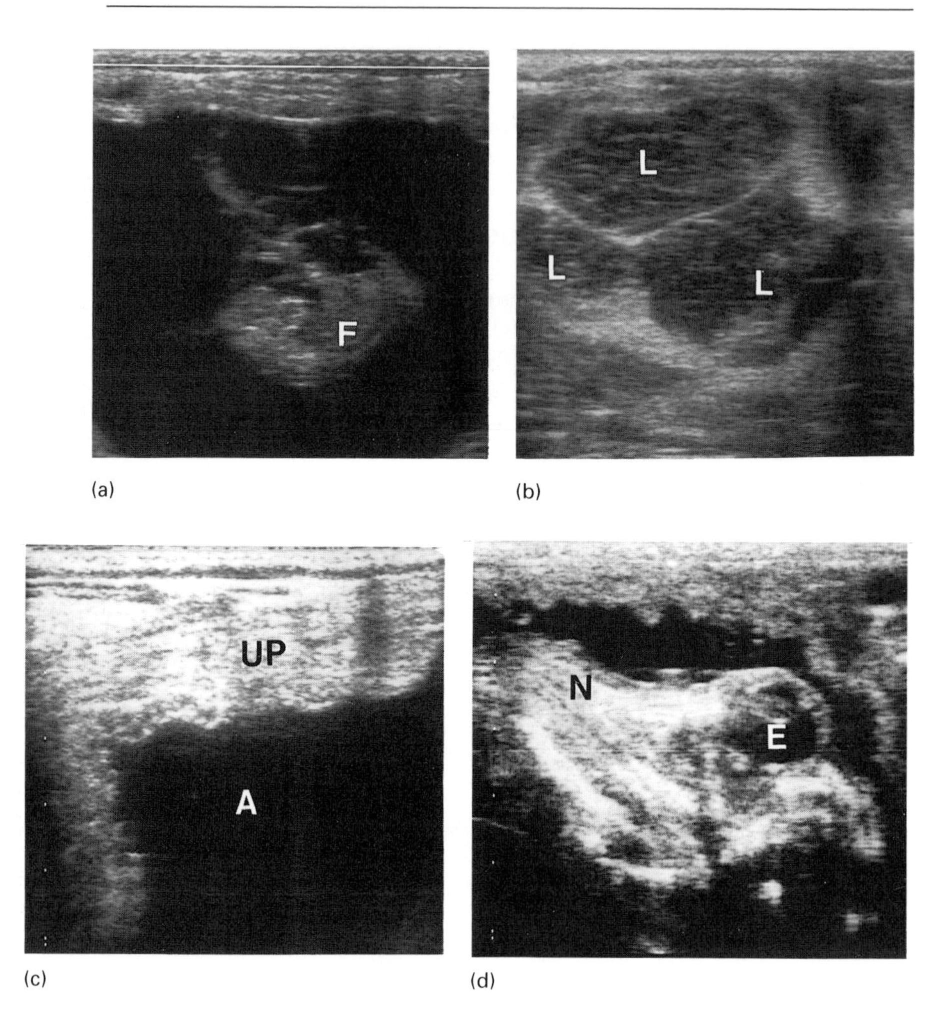

Fig. 8.2. Ultrasound images of equine pregnancy after day 40 (7.5 MHz transducer, scale in cm).
(a) Day 45 conceptus: differentiation of the fetus (F) can be readily identified. (b) Equine chorionic gonadotrophin stimulates secondary follicles to luteinise (L) from approximately day 45 onwards. (c) The fetus moves to a ventral position and may not be visible. It is possible to identify the uterine wall and placenta (UP), and the allantoic fluid (A). (d) Anechoic fetal eye (E) at 110 days of pregnancy; the nasal bones (N) can be clearly seen.

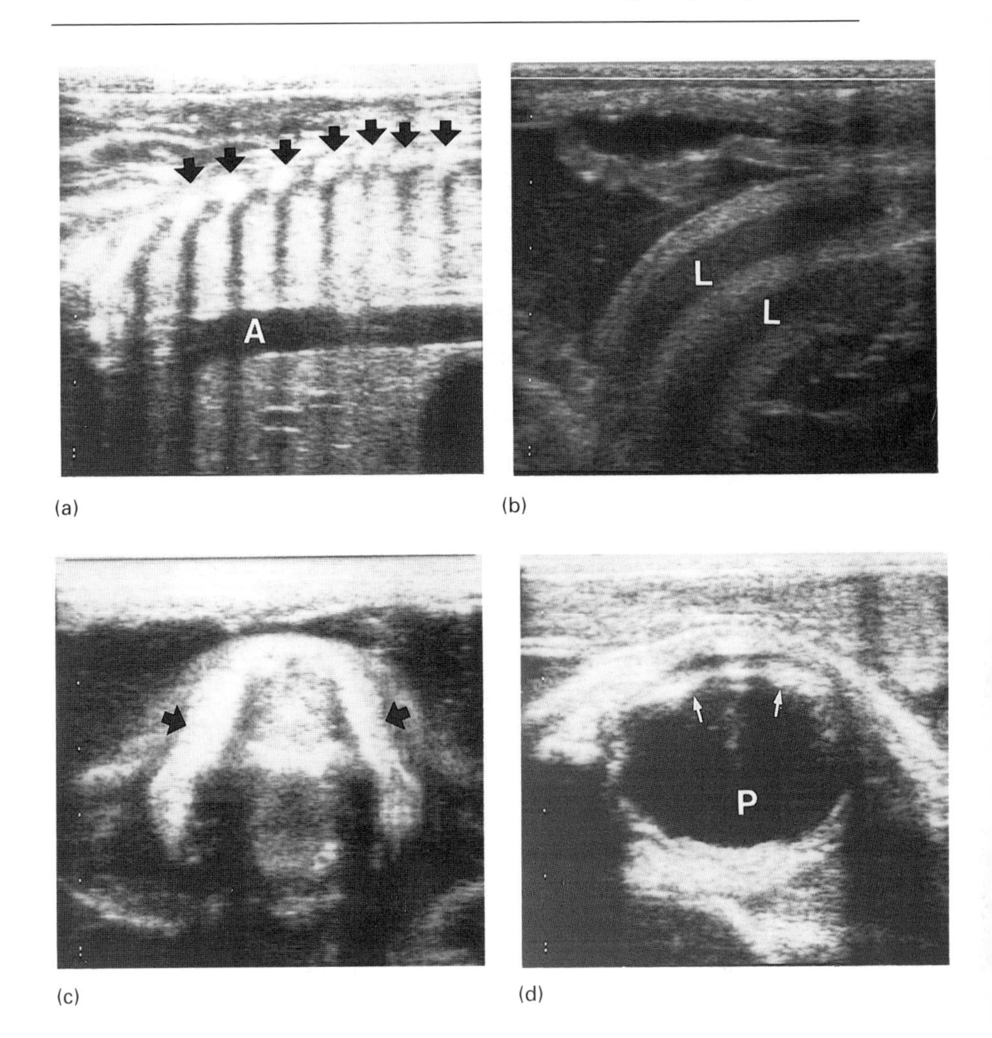

Fig. 8.3. Ultrasound images of late equine pregnancy (7.5 MHz transducer, scale in cm).
(a) Fetal thorax: the aorta (A) can be seen; shadowing artifacts are produced by ribs (arrows). (b) Two tubular structures representing a portion of the umbilical cord in longitudinal section: the central lumen (L) which is blood filled and therefore anechoic can be easily seen. (c) Transverse image of the rostral head demonstrating the nasal bones (arrows). (d) Sagittal section through fetal eye: the posterior chamber (P) can be imaged caudal to the iris (arrows).

imaged and the fetus may be seen by using a lower frequency transducer either transrectally or transabdominally.
- From 8 months of pregnancy it may be difficult to image more than a small portion of the fetus because of its large size.
- In the last trimester the amniotic cavity is increased in volume and the amniotic fluid contains multiple small echogenic particles.

8.7 TIME OF ULTRASOUND EXAMINATIONS FOR PREGNANCY

First examination at day 14–16

- The aim is to diagnose pregnancy and to ensure that the pregnancy is a singleton.
- The conceptus is spherical and anechoic with a dorsal and ventral specular echo.
- Examine the ovaries and count the number of luteal structures (multiple conceptuses nearly always originate from separate ovulations, and therefore result in multiple luteal structures).
- Multiple conceptuses may lie adjacent to each other or be separate.
- Conceptuses are mobile and careful examination of the entire tract is necessary to identify them.
- If multiple conceptuses are identified they can be managed since they are not fixed in position until after day 16.
- Multiple conceptuses can be separated and the smaller one crushed (see **20.3**).
- The mare should be examined 2 to 3 days later if a twin has been crushed.

Second examination at day 21–22

- The aim is to confirm the diagnosis of pregnancy, ensure that the pregnancy is a singleton and monitor the growth of the conceptus.
- Conceptus is fixed at base of one uterine horn.
- The conceptus can be distinguished from a uterine cyst by the presence of an embryo.
- Identification of a heart beat confirms embryonic viability.

Third examination at day 35

- The aim is to confirm the diagnosis of pregnancy, to monitor viability of the conceptus and to make any final decision before formation of the endometrial cups and the secretion of equine chorionic gonadotrophin (see pseudopregnancy **17.5**, **19.4**).

8.8 PROTOCOL FOR ULTRASOUND EXAMINATION

First examination at day 14–16

- If there is no suspicion of multiple conceptuses (single ovulation; single corpus luteum):
  (1) single conceptus imaged → re-examine at day 21
  (2) no conceptus imaged → check ovulation date; if correct inject PG, if uncertain re-examine in two days.
- If there is a suspicion of multiple conceptuses (multiple ovulations; multiple luteal structures):
  (1) single conceptus seen → re-examine in two days; if still single conceptus → re-examine at day 21
  (2) multiple conceptuses seen → PG
  → or, do not treat (little point as only 14 days pregnant)
  → or, crush the smaller conceptuses
  → re-examine in 2 days
  if single remains → re-examine at day 21
  if all concept uses lost → inject PG.

Second examination at day 21–22

- Expect to see increased size of conceptus.
- Anechoic yolk sac.
- Embryo (with heart beat) positioned at ventral pole.
- If these are not identified this may necessitate termination of the pregnancy using PG.

Third examination at day 35

- Expect to see small volume yolk sac, with embryo at the dorsal pole.
- Large volume of allantois.
- The amnion may also be imaged.
- Last time for interferences before endometrial cups secrete eCG.

8.9 DIAGNOSIS OF FETAL SEX

Fetal sex may be accurately diagnosed between 65 and 90 days after ovulation.

- Interpretation is difficult unless the operator is experienced.
- Diagnosis relies upon identifying the position and appearance of the genital tubercle.
- Care must be taken to differentiate the umbilicus accurately.

8.10 UTERINE CYSTS – STRUCTURES THAT MAY MIMIC PREGNANCY (Fig. 8.4)

Endometrial glandular or lymphatic cysts are not uncommon in the mare. They are fluid filled and therefore appear anechoic when imaged with ultrasound.

- Cysts commonly have a fine moderately echogenic wall which may not be fully appreciated unless there are multiple cysts or there is free uterine fluid.
- Cysts may range from several millimetres to several centimetres in diameter.
- Luminal cysts may be confused with early conceptuses.

To avoid these problems it is prudent to record the size, shape and position of uterine cysts prior to breeding (at the first ultrasound examination of the year); cysts do change in their appearance during the year; however, their position is constant. If a cyst has not previously been mapped it may be diagnosed as a cyst because:

- cysts are often irregular in outline
- cysts are frequently lobulated
- cysts do not always have dorsal and ventral pole specular echoes
- cysts do not change position
- cysts do not increase in size
- large cysts do not contain an embryo, whilst this can be seen in a conceptus after day 21.

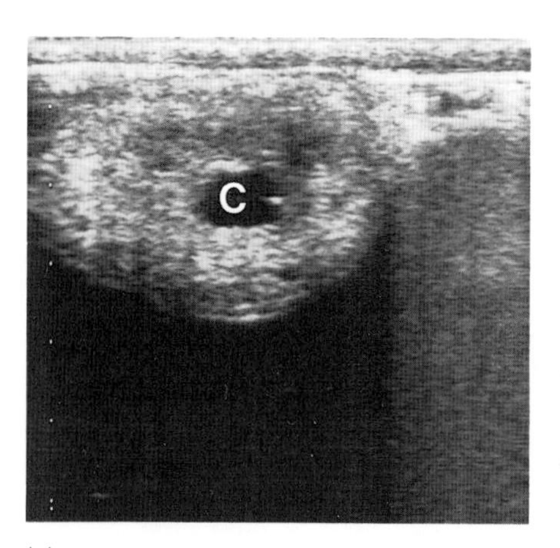

(a)

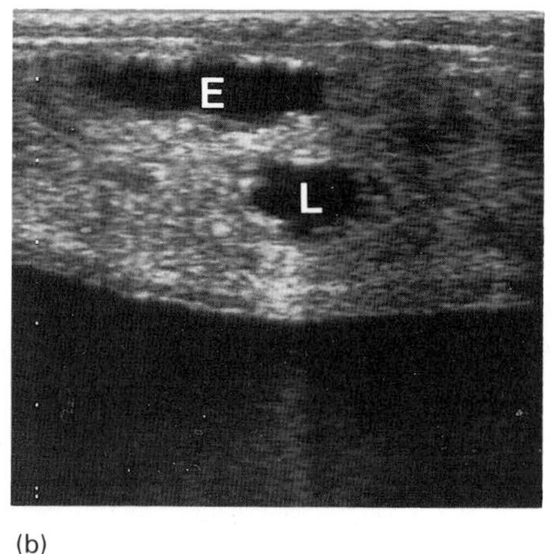

(b)

Fig. 8.4. Ultrasound images of endometrial cysts (7.5 MHz transducer, scale in cm).
(a) Central anechoic luminal cyst (C) present within the uterine horn.
(b) Luminal (L) and extraluminal (E) cysts present within the uterine body.

9 Normal Parturition

9.1 ENDOCRINE CONTROL

Parturition is rapid in the mare and the endocrine control is poorly understood. It is clear, however, that the changes are dissimilar to those observed in many other domestic animal species.

Progesterone

- Progesterone concentrations are low in the third trimester of pregnancy.
- Progesterone concentrations show a rapid rise in the last 30 days of pregnancy.
- Progesterone concentrations peak 2–3 days before parturition and decline after parturition.
- These changes are unlike other domestic species.

Oestrogen

- Oestrogen concentrations do not increase prior to parturition.
- The mare therefore undergoes a change in the progesterone:oestrogen ratio.

Relaxin and Prolactin

- There is a slight increase in relaxin during parturition.
- There is no large pre-partum surge in prolactin, unlike that seen in other domestic species.

Prostaglandin

- A gradual increase in the prostaglandin metabolite occurs in the last few months before parturition.
- It has been proposed that the site of prostaglandin production is the feto-placental unit.

9.2 PREPARATION OF THE ENVIRONMENT

1 Mares probably foal most naturally outside, but:

- constant surveillance is difficult
- other horses may molest the foal
- fetal membranes may be predated before inspection
- the foal may be damaged in wire and hedges, or drown in ponds and ditches, etc.

2 Mares foaling in boxes require:

- adequate room – a box at least 4 metres × 4 metres
- minimal disturbance
- good bedding – well compacted over concrete floor and built up at the walls
- minimal low-level feed bins; water bucket should be off the floor
- lots of time and patience.

9.3 THE 'OVERDUE' FOAL (7.8)

1 The biggest problem the foaling mare has is her owner, because:

- the owner expects foaling to occur 11 months after conception, and yet gestation length is very variable
- the owner does not understand that the mare will foal when she is ready, not when the owner thinks she is 'due'
- the owner has taken time off work to stay up at night to observe the foaling. He/she is now exhausted, must return to work and worry about the 'expectant mother'
- the owner suspects that an 'overdue' mare is harbouring a dead foal. Mares do not retain dead (single) foals; they are normally aborted
- the owner thinks the foal will be oversized if pregnancy is long. This is very unlikely because prolonged pregnancies usually indicate slow growth of the foal; fetal oversize is rare in horses, irrespective of parent size
- the owner has planned a party to coincide with foaling. Mares need minimal disturbance during parturition, and interference can cause the mare to delay expulsion and might result in dystocia.
- celebrate nothing until the foal is at least one week old!

2 In the event of a mare not foaling at the expected time, the Veterinary Surgeon may:

- examine the mare *per rectum* to confirm that she is pregnant
- confirm, by feeling fetal movement, that the foal is alive (to reassure the owner)

- confirm, if palpation of the foal's head is possible, that it is in an anterior presentation
- possibly, examine the cervix *per vaginam* for evidence of relaxation and liquification of cervical mucus. The cervix in late pregnancy is normally very soft, the canal is only $\frac{1}{2}$–1 cm long. The fetus is often palpable *per vaginam*.
- pre-partum the cervical mucus is very tacky; repeated examinations are not recommended.
- check that the expected foaling date has been calculated correctly.

9.4 FIRST STAGE PARTURITION

This is defined as commencing at the onset of uterine contractions.

- The beginning of first stage cannot be recognised.
- This is the preparation for the expulsive (second) stage.
- The mare is restless, looks at her flanks and shifts her weight from one hind limb to another (these signs can also be seen for months before foaling).
- Slackening of the sacro-sciatic ligaments and relaxation of the vulva are inconsistent signs.
- The escape of a honey-like precursor of colostrum (wax), onto the ends of the teats is a good sign that the mare is in the 'first stage' – but some mares expel obvious milk for days before foaling and others never wax-up.
- There is a rise in the calcium and potassium content of udder secretion before foaling, and a fall in sodium; the concentrations of potassium and sodium become similar (about 40 mmol/litre) 24–48 hours pre-partum.
- The signs of first stage parturition are basically those exhibited by a mare suffering myometrial contractions prior to opening of the cervix. The intensity of the signs depends on the mare and her environment.
- Mares in first stage parturition may hold their breath and grunt, but they do not normally strain; this is explosive and expulsive and occurs during second stage.
- The cervix may be dilated and feet may be found presented in the vagina before the onset of the second stage.

9.5 SECOND STAGE PARTURITION, I.E. EXPULSION (see also Chapter 23)

This commences with the onset of abdominal contractions.

- The cervix opens relatively quickly to allow the separating CAM to bulge into the vagina (**7.3**).
- Eventually the pressure in the vagina causes either the CAM to rupture,

with the visible loss of allantoic fluid from the vulva, or the mare to strain.

- Either event marks the beginning of second stage labour and has evoked Ferguson's reflex, i.e. vaginal distension causes oxytocin release and further myometrial contractions; if the CAM hasn't ruptured, it does so now.
- Mare is usually in lateral recumbency.
- Straining involves tensing of abdominal muscles and rigidity of all four limbs.
- The amnion, a white glistening membrane, soon becomes visible at the vulva containing fluid and/or a fetal foot.
- Both front feet (one further forward than the other) and the nose should appear in quick succession.
- After expulsion of the head the mare may stand and even eat, or may roll to change the position of the foal.
- Further straining ensures delivery of the chest and hips.
- If left undisturbed, the mare may lie for some time with the foal's hind limbs in her vagina.
- The foal is born in the amnion, but ruptures this when it attempts to sit up.
- Movement of the dam or foal causes the umbilical cord to rupture close to the abdominal wall.
- The mare's instinct is to lick the foal dry, but not to eat the membranes.
- Second stage labour usually occurs at night, and lasts 5–25 (mean 15) minutes.

9.6 THIRD STAGE PARTURITION (EXPULSION OF THE MEMBRANES)

Expulsion of the fetal membranes has usually occurred within three hours.

- The mare may show signs of abdominal pain due to continued uterine contractions.
- The weight of the amnion gently pulling on the CAM via the umbilical cord causes separation.
- The CAM is turned inside out during expulsion (Fig. 9.1).
- The membranes should be kept and inspected to ensure that they are complete (**21.2**).

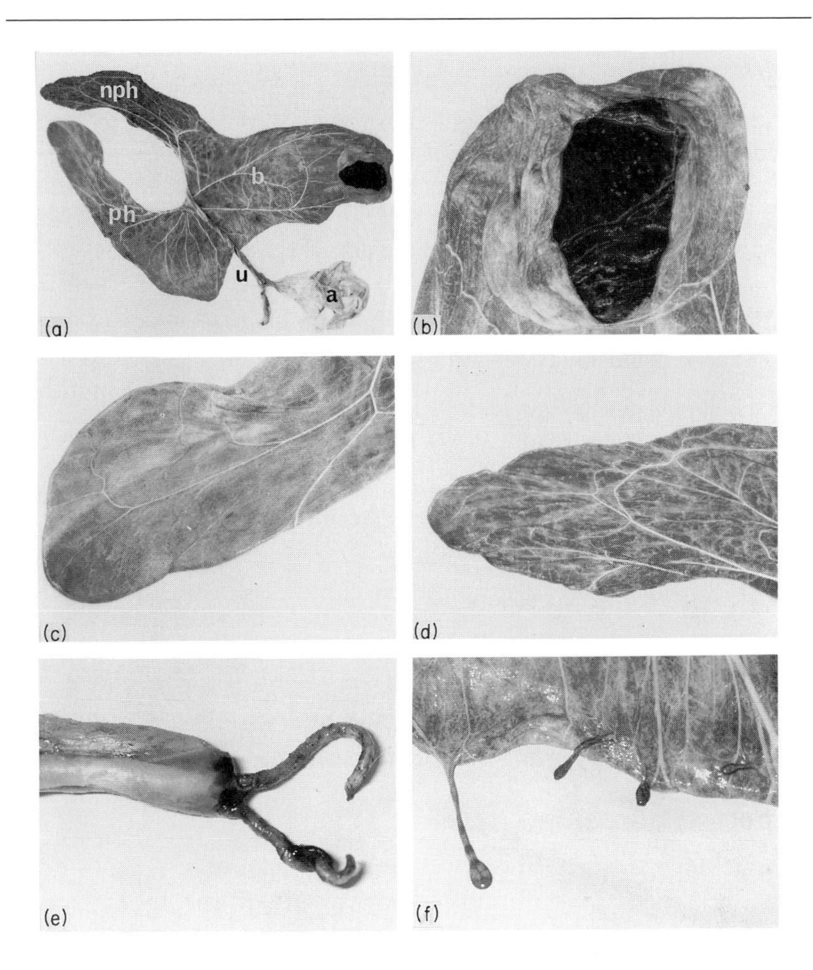

Fig. 9.1. Fetal membranes. (a) Complete set of fetal membranes showing the amnion **a**, umbilical cord **u** and the inner surface of the chorio-allantois **b** body; **ph**, pregnant horn; **nph**, non-pregnant horn. (b) Site where the allantochorion ruptured at the cervix. (c) Tip of pregnant horn (oedematous). (d) Tip of non-pregnant horn. (e) End of umbilical cord showing the umbilical arteries which ruptured within the foal's abdomen. (f) Chorio-allantoic vesicles containing the remnants of the endometrial cups.

9.7 INDUCTION OF PARTURITION

Indications

- Rarely necessary because long pregnancies are physiological and fetal oversize is not a problem.
- Useful in a very uncomfortable mare running milk with ventral oedema and relaxation of the cervix.

Criteria for induction

- Adequate gestation length, i.e. in excess of 320 days, although most Veterinary Surgeons will not consider induction until well past this time.
- Adequate mammary development, preferably with milk.
- The mare may be pre-treated with oestradiol, e.g. 5–10 mg 24 hours before attempting induction with the aim of relaxing the cervix.

Drugs used

1 Low dose oxytocin (10 IU) intravenously.

- Foaling begins within 15 to 30 minutes.
- Repeat administration at 20 minutes if parturition has not commenced.

2 High dose oxytocin (40 IU) intramuscularly.

- More discomfort to mare.
- Prolonged time to delivery.

3 Twice the luteolytic dose of prostaglandin.

- More effective the closer the mare is to term.
- Most mares undergo parturition within 4 hours.
- The interval to parturition may however be up to 56 hours.

Expected outcome

- Parturition may proceed normally within $1\frac{1}{2}$ hours.
- Initially, especially after oxytocin, the mare may be very uncomfortable and sweat profusely; this may be followed by a calm period before second stage parturition.
- Progress should be monitored by palpation of the cervix *per vaginam*.
- Repeat doses of either drug may be necessary.
- Expulsion of the foal may require assistance.
- Parturition may not be induced in some mares.
- Retrospectively, mares that foal most rapidly after induction are mares which were closest to their physiological foaling time.

Complications

- Veterinary Surgeon should remain close at hand once induction has started, although this may be expensive.
- Dystocia may occur due to inability or unwillingness of the foal to rotate during expulsion; this may be a sign of unreadiness for birth.
- The foal may be produced dead (suffocated) in the chorio-allantoic membrane.
- Immature and dysmature foals have trouble adapting to extra-uterine life and may die.

10 Post-partum Events

The mare is unusual compared with many other domestic species; uterine involution is extremely rapid, and there is a return to fertile oestrus within a few weeks of parturition. A new pregnancy may be established very early in the post-partum period.

10.1 UTERINE INVOLUTION

- Amazingly rapid after normal parturition.
- Histologically there is no disruption of the endometrium at parturition.
- The uterine horn which housed the fetus will remain larger than the other horn.
- It may be difficult to define when involution is complete, i.e. when the previously pregnant horn is no longer identifiable by palpation.
- The cervix remains relaxed until after the foal heat ovulation.
- New pregnancies almost invariably establish in the smaller uterine horn (previously non-gravid).
- There is uterine tone during involution and after the foal heat. This may make early manual diagnosis of pregnancy difficult; enlargement at the base of the previously pregnant horn may be mistaken for an 18–28 day conceptus.

10.2 ASSESSMENT OF UTERINE INVOLUTION

- Transrectal palpation may allow an estimation of the size of the uterus.
- Vaginal or speculum examination may allow inspection of the cervix and of any cervical discharge.
- Transrectal ultrasound examination allows accurate imaging of the uterus. The uterine dimensions, thickness of the uterine wall, presence of luminal fluid, and presence of luminal debris can be easily assessed.

10.3 POST-PARTUM INFECTION

- Bacteria may enter the mare's uterus post-partum.
- This can be reduced by immediately suturing or clipping the dorsal vulva closed after delivery.
- The post-partum uterine flora is usually dominated initially by coliforms, and later by β-haemolytic streptococci.
- Post-partum colonisation of the uterus by bacteria is a normal event, and it should be expected.
- After normal parturition, most mares eliminate bacteria before the foal heat.
- For the first few days after parturition there is a moderate vulval discharge (lochial fluid expelled from the uterus).
- Very little discharge is normally seen after the first few days post-partum.

10.4 ASSESSMENT OF POST-PARTUM INFECTION

- Post-partum infection of any significance is associated with uterine luminal fluid that can be detected using ultrasound imaging.
- Persistent vulvar (cervical) discharge is indicative of infection.
- Uterine swabs may be investigated for the presence of bacteria and/or neutrophils.

10.5 POST-PARTUM CYCLICITY

- Most mares usually return to oestrus approximately 5–9 days after parturition.
- This oestrus is generally known as the 'foal heat', since the foal often develops a physiological scour at this heat.
- Diarrhoea in the foal makes the identification of oestrus in the mare more obvious.
- Post-partum oestrus may not occur for a variety of reasons:
  (1) The mare foaled early in the year, or in adverse climatic conditions. The mare may therefore enter an effective seasonal anoestrus. In these cases cyclical activity will return when climatic conditions improve, the day length increases, and the mare's plane of nutrition is adequate.
  (2) The mare has normal endocrinological changes but is reluctant to exhibit oestrus due to maternal instinct. This is termed silent oestrus, and is related to the mare being protective of the foal. Silent oestrus in this instance may be prevented by either holding the foal securely near to the head of the mare, or confining it to a loose box away from the mare; the mare may need to have a twitch applied.

- Following the first post-partum oestrus the mare may also fail to cycle, this may be for a variety of reasons:

  (1) The mare continues to have silent oestrus.
  (2) The mare enters prolonged dioestrus (the corpus luteum persists).
  (3) The mare may enter anoestrus, although in this case it is more likely that the mare did not ovulate at the first post-partum oestrus.

- The fertility at the first post-partum oestrus has been recorded as being between 5 and 10% lower than at subsequent oestruses. This may be related to a failure of the uterus to become completely involuted; when ovulation occurs more than 10 days after parturition the pregnancy rate is higher than when ovulation occurs before day 10.
- Opinion as to whether the foal heat should be used or not is divided; each mare should be evaluated individually according to the following criteria:

  (1) Don't use foal heat if:

    - involution is physically poor (uterine fluid, thickened uterine wall detected with ultrasound)
    - the mare has a discharge or a positive culture (or neutrophils) at mating time (**14.3**)
    - the mare had dystocia or retained fetal membranes (**21.3**)
    - the mare foaled early and an even earlier foal is not required
    - if the mare has ovulated by the eighth day post-partum or earlier she is unlikely to conceive.

  (2) Do use foal heat if:

    - the mare foaled late in season
    - post-partum events seem normal
    - involution is adequate (assessed by palpation and ultrasound examination)
    - the mare is known to have aberrant cycles after the foal heat.

  (3) Advantages of using the foal heat:

    - It is easily recognisable because of foal scour and the record of recent foaling.
    - It avoids the confusion of erratic cyclic behaviour thereafter.
    - It may be last chance of conception for late foalers.

  (4) Disadvantages of using foal heat:

    - Conception rate is lower than for other heats.
    - Subsequent pregnancy loss may be higher.
    - Mating a mare with a diseased endometrium may prejudice against conception at a later heat or even cause permanent damage, especially after the first foal.

11 Normal Expectations of Fertility

11.1 CONCEPTION AND FOALING RATES

Horses have always been selected for breeding by man on the basis of their performance or conformation, i.e. they have never been selected for fertility.

- Horses are relatively infertile when compared with native ponies and other domesticated species because:

  (1) seminal quality is very variable among stallions and
  (2) many mares exhibit erratic and unpredictable reproductive behaviour.

- Pregnancy rates at any one heat may vary from 40–70% in large breeds of horse; this value is generally higher for ponies.
- Some apparently normal mares require mating at up to four heats to become pregnant; others fail to conceive until the next season.
- Overall pregnancy rates at the end of the season vary between 50% and 90%, and this depends upon:

  (1) fertility of the stallion
  (2) fertility of the mares
  (3) value of the horses involved, i.e. intensive veterinary management of mares where cost warrants this, results in better fertility *and* very expensive stallions do not usually attract mares which have low fertility.

- Pregnancy loss, after confirmed conception, is about 15%; this figure is lower for ponies (**17.2**, **17.4**).
- Horse breeding at any level is a gamble because you may not get a foal, or the foal you do get may not be the one you want.

11.2 EFFECT OF MANAGEMENT ON FERTILITY

- Most stallion owners want maximal fertility for their horses because this is their best form of advertising.

- Running a stud is a compromise between the expectations of the mare owners, the quality of the mares, the money involved and the expected value of the foals.
- Good studs tease mares regularly and individually; this involves the employment of sufficient trained staff.
- Mare owners who want to transport their mare to the stallion when in heat must be aware that the mare may have fooled them, and that recently travelled mares may not be relaxed enough to accept service.
- Many mares which arrive at stud said by their owners to be in heat are not.
- Mares fail to exhibit heat for many reasons (**12.1**, **12.2**, **12.4**); this may be a management fault, but is more often a problem of the mare.
- The length of time for which a mare fails to show heat before veterinary advice is sought depends on the policy of the stud and the attitude of the owner.
- Such a decision should involve consideration of:

  (1) the cost of veterinary treatment
  (2) the cost of keeping a mare at stud
  (3) the stage of the breeding season.

- Veterinary attention to a brood mare may be of benefit to three different factions:

  (1) The stud in general, e.g. swabbing for venereal diseases (**14.1**) and post-mortem examination of aborted fetuses and dead foals, i.e. identification of specific diseases, allows measures to be taken to prevent spread.
  (2) The mare owner, e.g. examination and treatment of mares not seen in heat, pregnancy diagnosis, treatment of mares with endometritis (**13.2**), and examination of mares which repeatedly fail to hold to service.
  (3) The stud owner, e.g. examination to ascertain the time of ovulation so that the mare only needs to be mated on a limited number of occasions; if the stallion has a lot of mares booked to him (i.e. is popular) this procedure is necessary to facilitate organisation of an efficient mating programme.

- Mistakes made by mare owners which contribute to poor fertility include:

  (1) presenting the mare for one day when she is thought to be in season
  (2) taking the mare home after mating and assuming that failure to observe subsequent heat is a reliable indicator of pregnancy
  (3) not allowing the stud owner to request reasonable veterinary attention to the mare
  (4) presenting a mare to stud late in the breeding season on a whim or due to a leg injury which precludes other use.

11.3 METHODS OF INVESTIGATING REPRODUCTIVE FUNCTION IN MARES

- Visual examination of the mare for general health, udder development and perineal conformation.
- Manual examination of the tract *per rectum* to assess reproductive status and diagnose pregnancy.
- Real-time ultrasound examination *per rectum* to assess reproductive status.
- Real-time ultrasound examination *per rectum* to anticipate the time of ovulation.
- Real-time ultrasound examination *per rectum* to diagnose post-mating endometritis.
- Real-time ultrasound examination *per rectum* to assess the response of endometritis to treatment.
- Real-time ultrasound examination *per rectum* to diagnose pregnancy and examine for twins.
- Real-time ultrasound examination *per rectum* to facilitate twin reduction.
- Manual examination *per vaginam* to assess reproductive status and identify lesions.
- Speculum examination *per vaginam* to assess reproductive status and collect cervical/uterine swabs.
- Swabbing uterus (via speculum or manually) to provide material for bacteriological culture and cytological examination.
- Biopsy of the uterus to provide a prognosis for mare's future breeding potential.
- Endoscopic examination of the uterus to identify lesions.
- Swabs from clitoris to identify carriers of venereal disease.
- Blood sampling for hormone analysis to (a) confirm mare's reproductive status and (b) pregnancy diagnosis.
- Blood sampling for chromosome analysis in mares which fail to mature sexually.

11.4 MANAGEMENT OF THE MARE AT STUD

There are many ways in which mares may be managed upon a stud (**11.2**). The method chosen depends upon the Veterinary Surgeon's experience and Stud Manager's ability.

Extensive management

- Veterinary Surgeon visits weekly or twice weekly.
- Mares teased daily.
- Mares mated every 48 hours until the end of oestrus.

Intensive management

- Veterinary Surgeon visits stud daily or every other day.
- Teasing uncommon.
- Mares examined repeatedly and cycles manipulated.
- Mares mated once during each cycle at an appropriate time in relation to ovulation.

The intensive management system has several advantages and disadvantages:

- Improved knowledge of stage of the cycle.
- More accurate timing of mating.
- Improved rate of conception to first service.
- Mare gets pregnant sooner and spends less time at stud.
- More efficient use of the stallion.
- More efficient detection of abnormalities; these can be dealt with rapidly.
- Academically more interesting for the Veterinary Surgeon.
- Increased cost, but this may be similar if the mare is managed extensively and does not get pregnant at the first mating.

12 Non-infectious Infertility in Mares

12.1 PROLONGED DIOESTRUS (4.9)

1 Caused by persistence of CL in absence of pregnancy.

- The CL can persist for up to three or more months.
- Not always related to early pregnancy loss, as it commonly occurs in mares which have never been mated.
- May occur after up to 25% of ovulations, i.e. it is common.
- CL is not palpable in ovaries, but follicles of various sizes develop, multiple follicles of up to 4 cm in diameter are common.
- Rarely one of these follicles ovulates to form a secondary CL; usually large follicles remain static or slowly regress.
- The uterus usually becomes firm and tubular (tonic) due to persistent progesterone stimulation from the CL.
- The cervix is typical of late dioestrus and early pregnancy.

2 Signs are failure to return to oestrus, especially during the breeding season, i.e. after an ovulation.
3 Treatment is by prostaglandin administration, which causes luteolysis and a return to oestrus in 3–5 days (and ovulation in 7–10 days).
4 One dose is usually sufficient but repeated doses may be needed because:

- mare may have had a dioestrus ovulation and the young CL (under five days) will not respond to prostaglandin
- there may be a large pre-ovulatory follicle in the ovary at the time of prostaglandin administration. The rapid decrease in progesterone after luteolysis allows quick ovulation without signs of oestrus and a new luteal phase begins; when a large follicle is palpated before prostaglandin administration, the mare should be teased daily thereafter and covered immediately she shows signs of heat. Some large follicles regress, however, and subsequent ovulation is from a new one; this can't be anticipated.

12.2 ERRATIC BEHAVIOUR EARLY IN THE SEASON (4.2)

This occurs early in the spring during the vernal transition.

1 Caused by mare trying, but failing, to produce ovulatory follicles.

- Sequential examination of the ovaries reveals waves of follicular development and regression.
- Follicles may reach a large size (4 cm) but fail to ovulate.
- Often multiple follicles are found within the ovaries.
- Single examinations can be confusing.
- It is difficult to predict the time of the ovulatory oestrus.
- The uterus is usually thin walled upon palpation.
- The cervix varies between typically anoestrus to that of early oestrus.

2 Signs are erratic oestrous behaviour of varied intensity, usually causing total confusion. The mare may accept mating for many weeks.

3 Treatment at this stage may be of little avail but should be along the following lines for avoidance (**5.1**):

- house and feed mare for at least two months before mating is expected. For mares to be mated from late April onwards this is not necessary
- subject the mare to 16 hours of 'good' light per day
- administer progestogens either orally or via an intravaginal device daily for 14–16 days. Follicular growth will occur and ovulatory oestrus should result soon after withdrawal of the drug
- ensure that lighting and housing routines are continued after the mare has gone to stud.
- There are no drug regimes applicable to clinical practice which will stimulate a mare in deep or shallow anoestrus to come into heat.

12.3 ERRATIC POST-PARTUM BEHAVIOUR (10.5)

1 Failure to show the 'foal heat', or failure to show oestrus thereafter may both occur.

- Mares may be having silent heats exhibiting a temporary true anoestrus, i.e. flaccid tract and inactive ovaries (**4.1**), or prolonged dioestrus.

2 Signs are failure to return to heat after foaling, or after the foal heat.

3 Treatment depends on cause:

- Anoestrus mares may respond to a course of progestogen.
- Mares with silent heat are treated as below.
- Mares with prolonged dioestrus respond to prostaglandin.

12.4 SILENT HEAT

1 A mare that will either not show signs of heat or will not allow mating, although rectal and vaginal examinations confirm that she is in oestrus and is close to ovulation.

- Usually seen in maiden mares or mares with young foals at foot; however, even a mare which usually 'shows well' can occasionally be affected.
- Must be distinguished from prolonged dioestrus in which there is also follicular development (**4.3**, **4.9**), which may be pronounced.

2 A mare is difficult to mate when she is physiologically in oestrus.

- The mare should be restrained as described in **6.6**.
- The foal may be held in front of the mare or confined out of earshot.
- Artificial insemination, if permitted, may be the last resort.

12.5 SPLIT OESTRUS

- Mare fails to show heat for 1–2 days during the middle of an otherwise normal oestrus, i.e. follicle continues to develop and eventually ovulates.
- Rarely diagnosed unless the mare is examined by palpation or using ultrasound as the initial cessation of oestrus is thought to indicate that ovulation has occurred.
- If recognised, the mare may be treated as for silent heat or return of normal behaviour may be awaited.

12.6 FAILURE OF CL FORMATION AFTER OVULATION

Evidence for the occurrence of this abnormality is scanty; if it does occur, it is most likely at the beginning and the end of the breeding season – haemorrhage may occur into an unruptured follicle with subsequent luteinisations (**12.7**).

12.7 LUTEINISED-HAEMORRHAGIC FOLLICLES

- Some follicles may reach ovulatory size but do not rupture.
- The oocyte is not released; therefore conception cannot occur.
- These changes can be identified with ultrasound (Fig. 12.1).
- Initially haemorrhage may occur into the follicle. This gives the appearance of small echogenic spots which float within the normally anechoic follicular fluid.

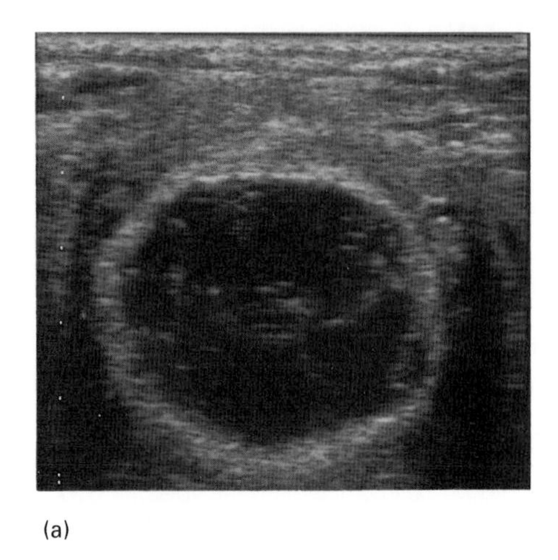

(a)

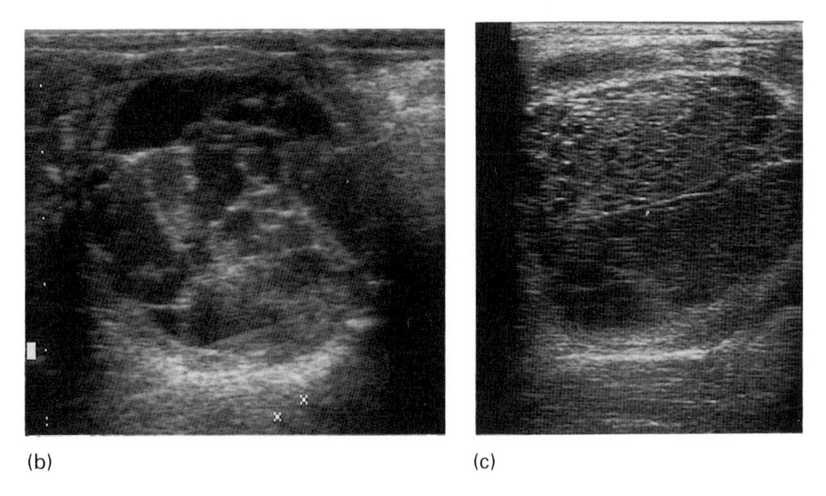

(b) (c)

Fig. 12.1. Ultrasound images of three different haemorrhagic-luteinised follicles (7.5 MHz transducer, scale in cm).
(a) Initial appearance of increased echogenicity within the follicular fluid associated with haemorrhage. (b) Three days after initial haemorrhage, extensive moderately echogenic tissue criss-crosses the follicular cavity. (c) Progressive luteinisation of the follicle observed with ageing of the structure.

- The echogenic regions coalesce and fine fibrin bands can be identified criss-crossing the follicle.
- The follicular cavity gradually increases in echogenicity associated with progressive luteinisation.
- Progesterone concentrations are elevated and the luteal phase is of an apparently normal duration.

- The resultant luteal structure is responsive to prostaglandin administration.

12.8 CYSTIC OVARIES DO NOT OCCUR IN MARES

- The term cystic ovaries implies the presence of large fluid filled structures which are either abnormal *per se*, or have developed in an abnormal manner.
- Such structures do occur in the ovaries of many animals, but *not* in the mare.
- Situations where 'cystic ovaries' are wrongly diagnosed in mares are as follows:

  (1) Mare's ovaries are large compared with those of cows and practitioners unfamiliar with this may misinterpret the normal mare ovary.
  (2) During the transition from anoestrus to regular cyclic behaviour there may be many persistent follicles in the ovaries (**4.2**, **12.2**); these are morphologically normal.
  (3) During prolonged dioestrus there is continued ovarian follicular activity not associated with heat – the ovaries are morphologically normal (**4.9**, **12.1**).
  (4) During early pregnancy there is massive and persistent ovarian activity (**7.6**); this also occurs in pseudopregnancy (**17.5**; **19.4**).

- Situations where cysts can be associated with mare ovaries (but *not* called cystic ovaries) are (Fig. 12.2):

  (1) Fossa cysts. These are found post-mortem in older mares and may be identified with ultrasound. They are very small (1–5 mm) and probably occur due to the developing CH enveloping a small amount of the fimbrial epithelium and dragging it into the ovary as the CL matures. Masses of cysts at the ovulation fossa could theoretically impeded ovulation.
  (2) Para-bursal cysts. These are remnants of the mesonephric tubules and are found in the mesovarium and mesosalpinx; they do not affect fertility.
  (3) Adrenocortical cysts. These are located within loose connective tissue covering the ovary; they do not affect fertility.

- Most cysts are usually not palpable. However, they may be imaged with ultrasound, and by the unwary may be confused with follicles or conceptuses. Careful examination allows identification of their position and therefore their nature.

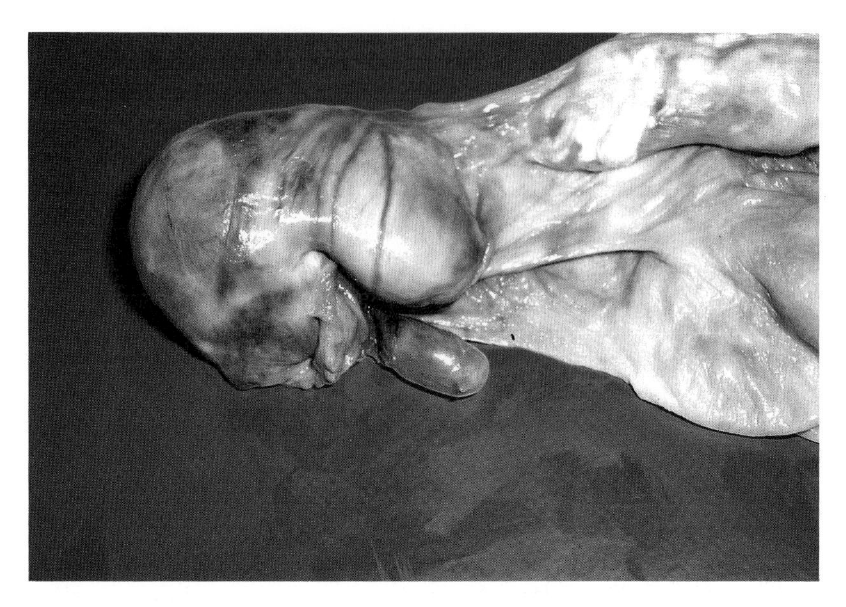

(a)

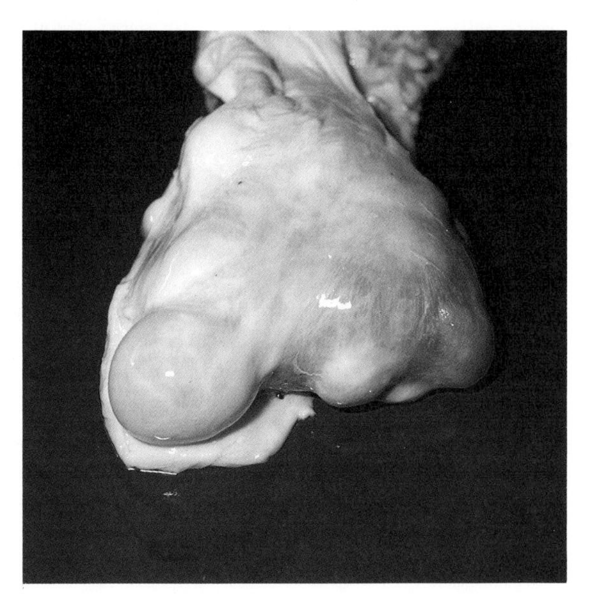

(b)

Fig. 12.2. (a) Fossa cyst: fluid filled thin walled structure noted adjacent to the ovulation fossa. (b) Para-bursal cyst: fluid filled thin walled structure present adjacent to the caudal pole of the ovary.

12.9 NYMPHOMANIA

True nymphomania probably doesn't exist in mares, but conditions which mimic it are:

- persistent oestrus during early spring. This is physiological and can be treated by trying to induce ovulation with hCG if a large follicle is present, or administering and withdrawing progestogens if many small follicles are present (**5.1**, **5.3**, **12.2**)
- mares which are bad tempered or otherwise difficult to handle during oestrus. Ovariectomy may give adequate control, but the likely outcome of this treatment can be tested by administering and withdrawing progestogen to abolish cyclical activity
- mares that are persistently vicious and difficult with other horses. They may squirt urine and 'show', especially when handled behind.These mares have normal ovaries and their problem is not sexual but psychological. Ovariectomy usually has no effect, but progestogen treatment can be tried as an indicator. Some response to the progestogen may, however, be the result of its central sedative action
- granulosa cell tumour (**12.10**).

12.10 GRANULOSA CELL TUMOUR

- This name is used to describe a family of histologically and endocrinologically different tumours (sex cord/stromal cell tumours) of the mare's ovary (other ovarian tumours are very rare).
- These tumours are often large before they are diagnosed. They often have a multiloculated appearance with thick divisions between individual cystic regions (Fig. 12.3).
- They can occur at any age, but usually affect young mares (5–9 years).
- Only one ovary is involved.
- Depending on the hormones that the tumour produces, the mare may show persistent anoestrus, persistent oestrus or virilism (male like behaviour).
- Diagnosis is by rectal examination of the ovary; this is large (8–30 cm diameter) spherical and hard, and the opposite ovary is usually small and inactive.
- Plasma concentrations of the steroid hormones may be elevated.
- Inhibin concentrations in plasma are usually markedly elevated.
- NB: Other ovarian conditions which may be confused with granulosa cell tumours are: large post-ovulation haematoma – this gradually becomes small over a period of weeks and a mare cycles normally; large active ovaries in spring, prolonged dioestrus, early pregnancy and pseudopregnancy type II – both ovaries are usually involved (**12.8**); teratoma – a very rare tumour of the ovary.
- Treatment is ovariectomy.
- The opposite ovary may take up to one year to resume normal function, and after this time the mare should cycle again.

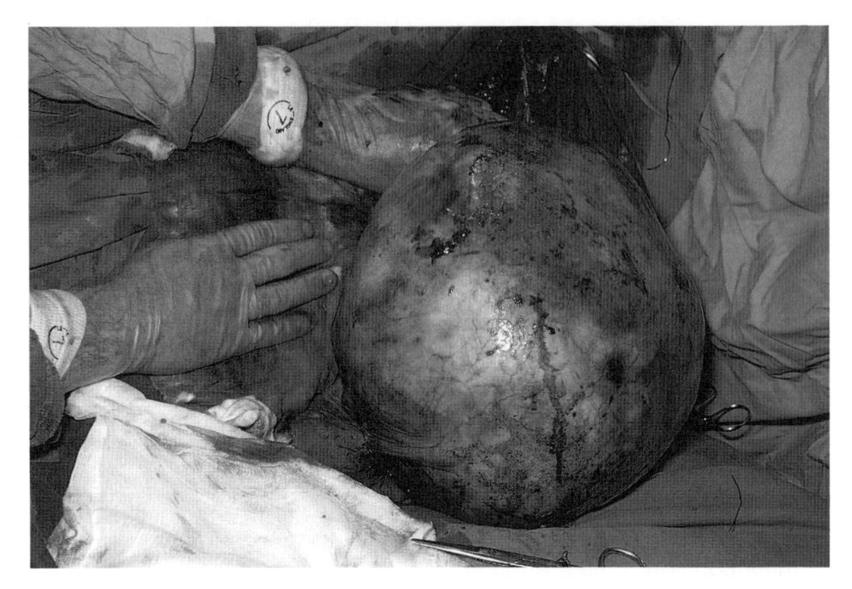

(a)

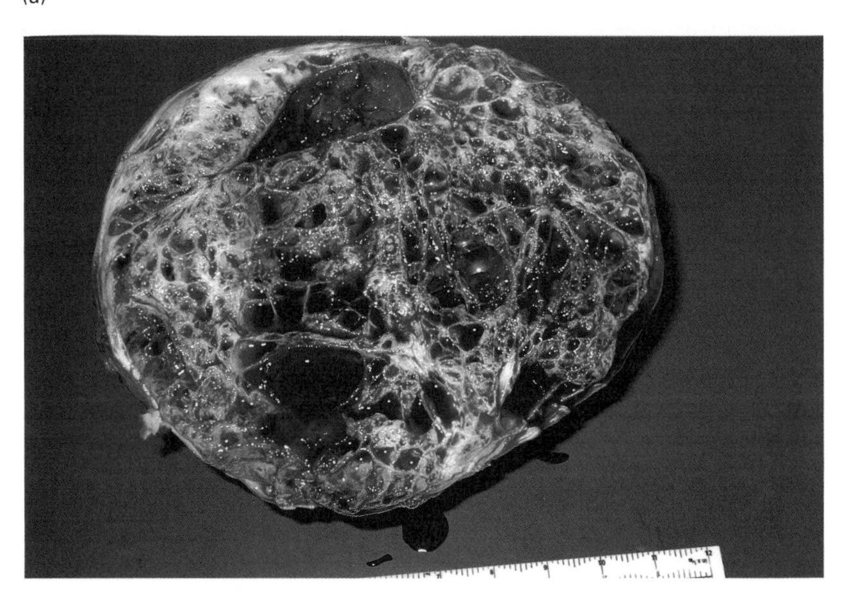

(b)

Fig. 12.3. (a) Surgical removal of large granulosa cell tumour. (b) Cut section of a granulosa cell tumour demonstrating its multiloculated appearance with thick fibrous divisions between individual fluid-filled regions.

12.11 CHROMOSOME ABNORMALITIES

Turner's syndrome (63, XO)

- Uncommon chromosomal abnormality which renders the mare sterile.
- Mares are usually small for their age and do not exhibit normal oestrous behaviour.
- Ovaries are very small and non-functional, and the uterus is thin-walled and difficult to palpate.
- Blood collection and karyotype examination will confirm the diagnosis.
- Some fillies out of training, even at 4 years, may have a quiescent reproductive tract, and need more time to mature (**2.4**).

Intersex

- Uncommon condition.
- Foal is thought to be a filly until puberty at which time the clitoris enlarges and becomes phallus like, urination occurs in an upwards direction and the filly exhibits male-like behaviour.
- The ano-genital distance may be large.
- Treatment is surgical removal of the gonads, which are usually testes and are intra-abdominal; surgery to the clitoris (phallus) may also be necessary with uncertain results.
- These animals may have abnormalities of chromosomal sex (chimeras), or abnormalities of gonadal sex (XX sex reversal).

Other chromosome abnormalities

- Recent investigations have shown that some mares which have primary infertility and gonadal hypoplasia have some identifiable chromosome abnormality.
- Some mares appear normal externally but have a hypoplastic reproductive tract; the commonest chromosome abnormality is 64, XY sex reversal.
- Some mares have normal external and internal genitalia but poor fertility; these include mares with abnormalities of chromosomal structure with rearrangement of genetic material (commonly balanced translocations).

12.12 ABNORMALITIES OF THE UTERINE TUBES

- This is very rare in mares, and when they do occur they are unlikely to be diagnosed ante-mortem.
- Abnormalities include adhesions, blockage and hydrosalpinx.
- Some practitioners may surgically flush the uterine tubes in the belief that they are blocked; one study, however, showed that 97% of 2000 pairs were patent.

12.13 UTERINE CYSTS

Uterine cysts are commonly identified with ultrasound imaging of the reproductive tract. The diagnosis of uterine cysts may or may not have significance for fertility; however, they must be correctly diagnosed and not confused with a pregnancy.

- Cysts are often small (less than 1 cm) but they may be extremely large (5 cm).
- Only large cysts can be diagnosed by palpation.
- Cysts are often present in small numbers, frequently clustered close to each other.
- Cysts may be conveniently categorised as being either luminal or extra-luminal.
- Smaller cysts are often luminal and generally originate from the uterine glandular tissue.
- Larger cysts are often extra-luminal and generally form from obstructed lymphatic channels.
- Ultrasonographically they appear as anechoic structures with a thin irregularly marginated wall.
- Luminal cysts are frequently pedunculated and have a wide-based attachment (Fig. 12.4).

There has been considerable debate about the significance of uterine cysts in relation to fertility. Generally:

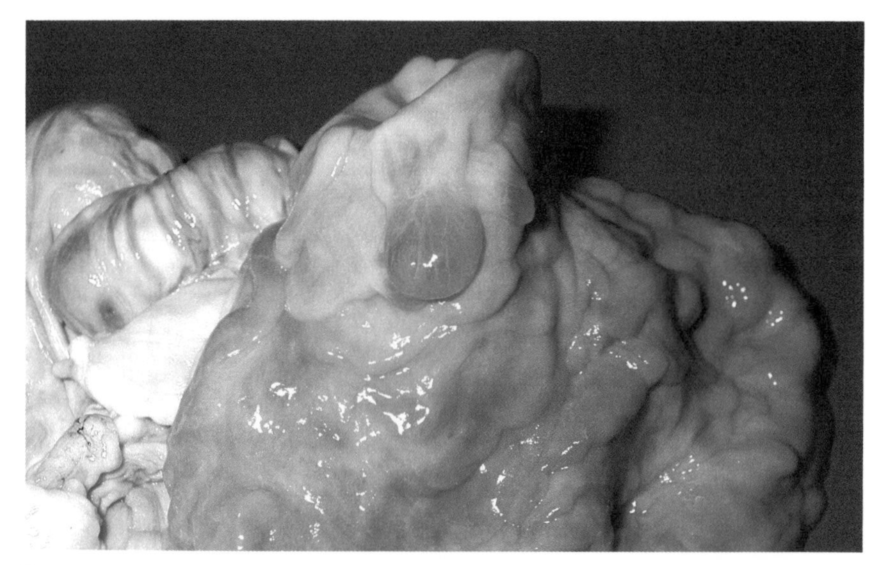

Fig. 12.4. Thin walled endometrial cyst filled with red-tinged fluid, present within the uterine body. In this view the uterus has been everted, and it can be clearly seen that this is a luminal cyst with a wide based attachment.

- Small endometrial cysts are of no clinical significance
- large cysts or an accumulation of smaller cysts in a single area may prevent the mobility phase of the conceptus and therefore result in a failure of maternal recognition of pregnancy; the corpus luteum is lost despite the presence of a conceptus and the mare returns to oestrus at an interval of approximately 21 days
- mares with numerous cysts may have an increased risk of embryonic loss during early pregnancy
- multiple, usually small, cysts have been observed in mares with chronic infiltrative lymphocytic endometritis. In these cases the prognosis for fertility is hopeless.

The major concern for most Veterinary Surgeons is the problems posed by cysts when attempting to diagnose early pregnancy using ultrasound.

- Endometrial cysts may mimic the appearance of an early conceptus since they are fluid filled.
- 'Mapping' of the shape, size and position of uterine cysts early in the breeding season ensures that this problem does not occur.
- If the mare has not previously been examined cysts may be distinguished from a conceptus since:

  (1) cysts are frequently not spherical in outline
  (2) cysts are often irregularly marginated and have small outpouchings
  (3) cysts are usually consistent in their position and do not increase in size, unlike a conceptus.

12.14 PARTIAL DILATION OF THE UTERUS

- A permanent dilation at the base of one or (rarely) both uterine horns may be rarely diagnosed by palpation.
- This change is probably the result of repeated pregnancies, but histologically it is associated with lymphostasis in that area.
- Dilation is easiest to palpate when the mare is in oestrus, i.e. when the uterus is oedematous.
- Dilation may allow persistence of uterine secretions and semen after mating, predisposing to endometritis (**13.2**).
- Treatment is as for mares with poor uterine resistance (**15.2**).

12.15 LESIONS OF THE CERVIX

1 Fibrosis of the cervix is often seen in older mares; sometimes in old maiden mares.

- This may be due to trauma at foaling in some mares.
- The result is that the cervix relaxes only slightly when mare is in oestrus.

- If the cervix is very narrow most of the ejaculate may remain in the vagina after mating and be subsequently lost.
- The condition may be diagnosed by introducing a tubular vaginal speculum immediately after mating. Any remaining ejaculate may then be collected and immediately inseminated into the uterus.
- The condition predisposes to endometritis as normal post-mating exudate cannot escape.
- Mares which conceive in this manner do not have trouble foaling.
- Severe constriction of the cervical canal may contribute to the development of pyometra (**15.3**).

2 Adhesions of the cervix are seen as a result of trauma (mating or foaling) or persistent vaginitis, or endometritis.

- Adhesions may completely occlude the cervical canal.
- They may be broken down manually but usually recur; devices intended to remain in the canal to prevent this are not reliable.
- They can be corrected by constant digital breakdown whilst the mare is in oestrus over several cycles.
- Surgical correction is rarely attempted.
- Prognosis for fertility is poor.
- They may contribute to the development of pyometra (**15.3**).

12.16 PERSISTENT HYMEN

- Manual vaginal examination of maiden mares often reveals hymenal tissue at the vestibulo–vaginal junction; this breaks down easily with manual pressure.
- Occasionally the hymen is complete and at 2–3 years of age a glistening membrane is seen to bulge from the vulva when the filly lies down or urinates.
- Manual examination reveals abrupt occlusion of the vagina just anterior to the urethral opening.
- The hymen can be very tough and is ruptured by penetration with a finger, a guarded needle or blade, or by retracing the hymen to the vulva with forceps and incising it.
- Incision allows the escape of milky secretions which have accumulated cranial to the hymen; there may be some bleeding.
- The small incision is easily expanded using a finger and hand.
- Rarely there are numerous strands of tissue between the vestibule and the cervical area; these require extensive blunt dissection.

12.17 VAGINAL BLEEDING

- Bleeding from the vulva after a potentially traumatic incident, i.e. mating or foaling, requires further investigation (**6.7**, **22.4**).

- Spontaneous vaginal bleeding in non-pregnant mares is usually more obvious in the morning, probably because blood has accumulated in the vestibule whilst the mare was resting overnight. Haemorrhage occurs from varicose vessels in the remnants of the hymen usually at the dorsal vestibulo–vaginal junction. Treatment is ligation of these vessels under local or general anaesthesia.
- Spontaneous vaginal bleeding in the pregnant mare:
    (1) rarely may be due to placental separation and signifies that foaling/ abortion is imminent
    (2) usually occurs in late gestation from lesions similar to those in the non-pregnant mare. In this case no treatment is necessary and bleeding ceases post-partum.

13 Infectious Infertility

13.1 GENERAL CONSIDERATIONS

Infections of the mare's uterus are common and in certain circumstances are normal. In these cases inflammation is usually confined to the endometrium. Systemic illness is only associated with inflammation of the whole uterus, i.e. metritis; this is rare and only occurs post-partum.

- A transient endometritis occurs after a mare is mated and after she foals; this is a normal reaction to the foreign protein and bacteria which enter the uterus at this time and is normally resolved within 24 hours of service and within 6 days of foaling.
- This 'physiological' endometritis is confirmed by finding bacteria and inflammatory cells in the uterine lumen, but may not produce an obvious discharge.
- In nearly all cases endometritis can be diagnosed by identifying the presence of fluid within the uterine lumen using ultrasound. Fluid may be anechoic but frequently contains echogenic particles.
- Persistence of endometrial infection occurs when:

  (1) the normal uterine drainage mechanisms are impaired
  (2) the mare's resistance to normal genital bacteria is reduced
  (3) specific invasive venereal pathogens are present.

- Endometritis causes infertility by:

  (1) providing an unsuitable uterine environment for the development of the conceptus
  (2) causing premature lysis of the CL thus ensuring very early pregnancy failure. This is the important reason why 'dirty' mares fail to conceive and suggests that later pregnancy failures cannot be due to mares having endometritis at the time of mating
  (3) causing placentitis and possible bacteraemia or septicaemia of the fetus in late pregnancy; this stimulates abortion due to fetal stress or death.

13.2 NON-SPECIFIC INFECTIONS

These usually include normal commercial organisms that in normal circumstances do not produce disease.

- The vestibular and clitoral area of the mare normally has a harmless and constantly fluctuating bacterial population; the stallion's penis is colonised by similar organisms.
- Washing and disinfecting the genitalia before service can reduce the bacterial population but:

  (1) no treatment will completely sterilise either area
  (2) overuse of antiseptics is contraindicated because removal of the normal bacterial population allows resistant and potentially dangerous bacteria (especially *Pseudomonas* spp.) to proliferate.

- Contamination of the mare's uterus, which is where most of the ejaculate is deposited, is physiological. The debris and bacteria derive from the stallion's penis and the mare's vestibule and vulva.
- Elimination of these bacteria under normal circumstances is rapid (i.e. less than 24 hours) and effective, but two situations arise where this is not possible.

Pneumovagina (wind sucking) (15.5)

- Faulty conformation of the vulva and/or vestibulo-vaginal constriction allows the mare to aspirate air into the vagina.
- Aspiration is persistent and the vagina may be contaminated from the adjacent rectal excretions.
- Aspiration causes desiccation of the vaginal mucosa and predisposes to bacterial infection; this spreads forward to the cervix and uterus and causes a chronic endometritis.
- Recognition of the condition may be easy if the mare makes an obvious noise whilst walking.
- Some mares are insidious windsuckers and may only do so when relaxed or whilst shifting weight from one hind leg to another in a box.
- Diagnosis can therefore be difficult, but the presence of froth (air and mucus) in the vagina is pathognomonic.
- The identification of gas within the uterus (using ultrasound) also indicates vaginal gas has been aspirated into the uterus, i.e. the mare is likely to have abnormal conformation.
- Treatment is by Caslick's vulvoplasty (Fig. 13.1) which results in fusion of the dorsal vulval labia, thus reducing the size of the orifice to prevent pneumovagina.
- In cases of severe conformational abnormality an episioplasty or a perineal body transection (Pouret's operation; Fig. 13.2) may be warranted.

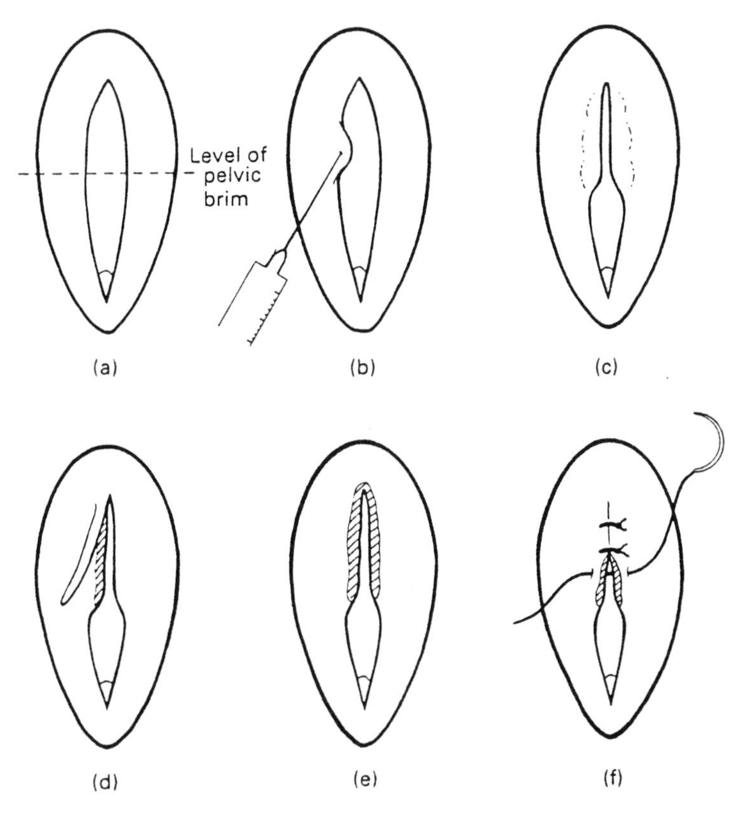

Fig. 13.1. Caslick's vulvoplasty. (a) After restraining the mare, clean her vulva and ascertain the level of the floor of the pelvis. (b) Starting at this level, infiltrate the mucocutaneous junction of the vulva with local anaesthetic (10–20 ml) through a 21 g l″ needle. (c) Infiltrate both sides up to the dorsal commisure. (d) Using rat toothed forceps and curved scissors cut a 2 mm strip of mucocutaneous junction from the anaesthetised area. (e) Ensure that tissue is removed completely from the dorsal commisure. (f) Coapt the cut areas with simple interrupted sutures or a blanket stitch.

Factors which predispose to pneumovagina

1 Negative intravaginal pressure; air can only enter the vagina if pressure there is less than atmospheric. This pressure difference is usually greater in horses than ponies, and pneumovagina is uncommon in ponies.
2 Damage to the vestibulo–vaginal junction, usually caused by over stretching; this can allow pneumovagina even though vulval conformation is normal.
3 Abnormal vulval conformation; normally the vulva slopes slightly forward and most of the length of its opening is below the level of the floor of the pelvis (ischium).

   Abnormal conformations include:

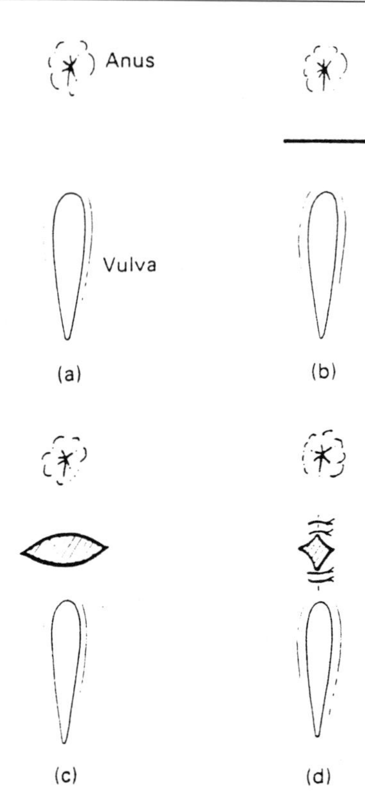

Fig. 13.2. Pouret's operation. (a) Induce epidural anaesthesia using about 10 ml of lignocaine (without adrenalin) in the sacro-coccygeal or first inter-coccygeal space. Clean the perineum. (b) Make a horizontal incision in the perineal body midway between the anus and vulva. (c) Bluntly dissect forward, without entering the rectum or vagina, to the retroperitoneal fat. Free the vagina laterally from its attachment to the pelvic wall. (d) Close the perineal skin converting the incision into a vertical one.

- underdevelopment and vertical positioning of the vulva in maidens, where more than half the orifice is dorsal to the ischium; this tends to cause pneumovagina in fillies in training
- horizontal vulva; due to ageing and weight loss (e.g. in winter) the anus sinks forward and pulls the vulva with it, so that part of the dorsal opening lies horizontally on the floor of the ischium. This not only predisposes to pneumovagina but allows gross contamination of the vestibule with faecal material
- tears of the vulval lips or scars which cause distortion (**22.1**).

4 Recto-vaginal fistula (**22.2**) and perineal laceration (**22.3**).

Caslick's vulvoplasty (Fig. 13.1)

1 Introduce antibiotic into the uterus as described later (**15.1**, **15.2**).

2 Clean the vulva with clean water and dry.

3 Ascertain the level to which the dorsal commissure of the vulva must be sutured; ideally this should be to the level of the ischial arch, but if conformation is very poor, i.e. the vulva is pulled dramatically forward, a compromise which allows just sufficient room for coitus should be reached (for severe perineal malformations episioplasty or perineal body transection should be considered). Alternatively the vulva is sutured to the ventral commissure, and is temporarily re-opened to allow mating.

4 After suitable restraint infiltrate the vulval lips with local anaesthetic:

- start at the most ventral point and use a small (23 g 1″) needle (Fig. 13.1)
- proceed dorsally stepwise, ensuring that the dorsal commisure is well infiltrated
- repeat on the other side
- for mares operated on previously, infiltrate deeply.

5 Using rat-toothed forceps and curved scissors cut a strip of mucosa at the mucocutaneous junction from the ventral limit of anaesthetised area to the dorsal commisure on both sides; ensure that the incision is complete dorsally and only remove mucosa. For mares that have been operated on previously, radical dissection may be necessary before healthy (bleeding) tissue is reached. For many mares a narrow strip (5 mm wide) is all that need be removed.

6 Suture one side of the vulva to the other using simple interrupted sutures or a locking pattern:

- suture material may be permanent or absorbable
- time of suture removal is not critical but must occur before the next foaling
- mares that require mating subsequently should be resutured immediately if ripping occurs; otherwise a deep mattress suture of tape, after deep local infiltration, should be inserted before mating (breeders stitch)
- sutured mares must be 'opened' with scissors just before parturition; if not the vulva may tear laterally causing shortening and deformity of the vulva
- tears of the vulva should be attended to immediately post-partum; in this case local anaesthesia may not be necessary. However, in the case of severe trauma, swelling, oedema or necrosis, it is prudent to allow at least 1 week before attempting repair. During this time a large amount of tissue may slough.

Impaired ability of the uterus to deal with infection

All mares develop a transient endometritis after mating. Normal mares can resolve this rapidly. Some mares are unable to deal with this endometritis and they are frequently termed 'susceptible' mares.

- Susceptible mares develop a persistent post-coital endometritis which persists and prevents the establishment of the pregnancy.
- The mare may conceive; however, pregnancy loss occurs when the conceptus reaches the uterus, or because of uterine prostaglandin production causing lysis of the corpus luteum.
- It was proposed that a local immune deficiency was the cause of this problem.
- Recently it has been suggested that uterine drainage is more important.
- Uterine drainage may be impaired in several circumstances:

  (1) failure of cervical relaxation associated with cervical fibrosis in older mares
  (2) cervical lesions including adhesions
  (3) impaired uterine contractility, especially in old mares and post-partum
  (4) high intravaginal pressure, such as that which occurs in mares with poor conformation, resulting in breakage of the vulval and vestibulo–vaginal seals, resulting in pneumovagina.

Diagnosis (recognition of the problem) is hampered by:

- ignorance of the fact that the condition exists
- failure of veterinary examination of the mare after mating
- failure to recognise the significance of a post-mating discharge from the vulva; some discharge is accepted as normal and it may be difficult to decide when this might be pathological
- most mares not being observed closely during the two weeks following the end of the heat; dioestrus discharge therefore goes unobserved.

Diagnosis

Accurate diagnosis of post-coital endometritis requires:

- ultrasonographic examination of the uterus 24 hours after mating. The presence of luminal fluid at this time should be considered to be highly suspect
- (collection of post-coital uterine swabs for bacteriological or cytological investigation)
- (careful clinical examination of the mare for the presence of any vulval (cervical) discharge)
- careful monitoring of the interval to the next oestrus since endometritis causes a shortening of the luteal phase and often a shortening of the total cycle to usually approximately 16 days but occasionally as short as 10 days; these mares may have an unobserved oestrus unless teasing is started before 17 days, and may then be considered to have had a long interoestrus period. If oestrus is detected at the heat after infection, discharge may be absent as a result of the following sequence of events:

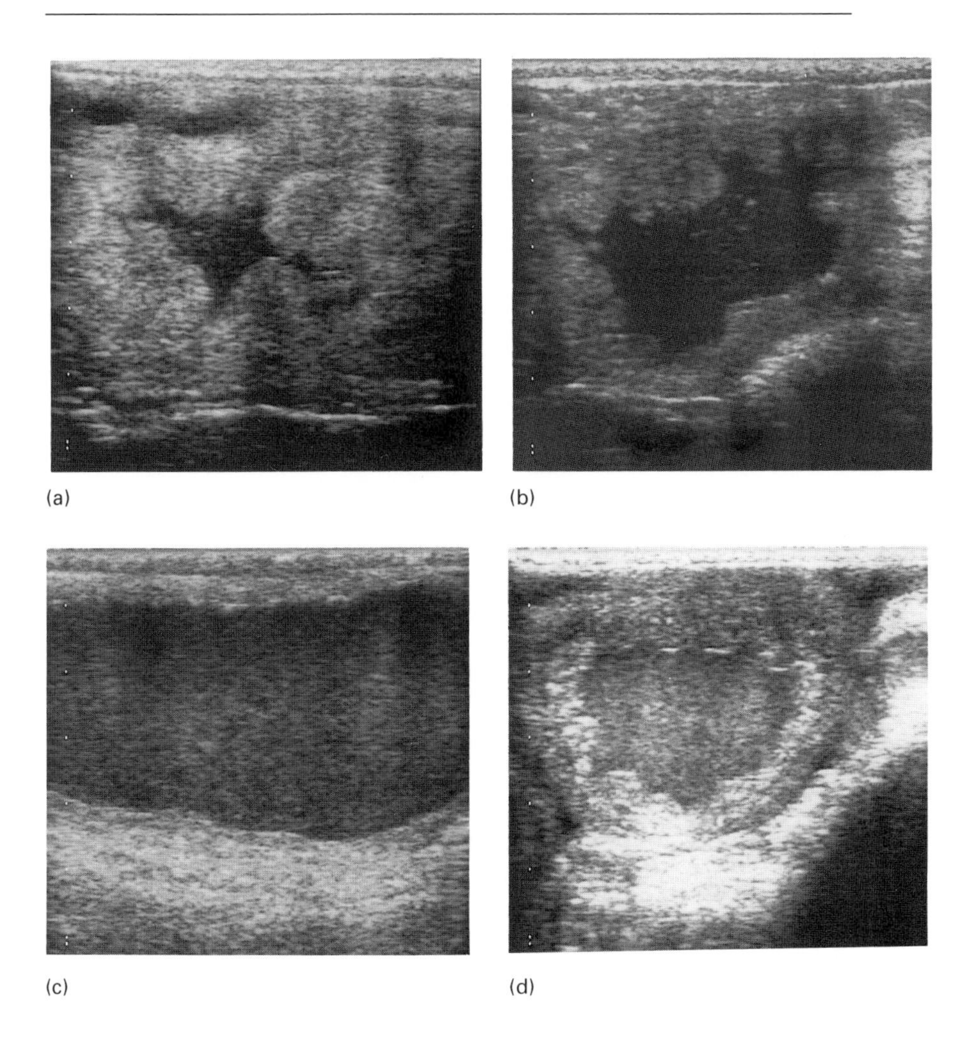

Fig. 13.3. Ultrasound images of mares with post-coital endometritis and pyometra (7.5 MHz transducer, scale in cm).
(a) Oedematous uterus with small volume of moderately hypoechoic luminal fluid 12 hours after mating. Neutrophils were present on an endometrial swab, although no bacteria were isolated. The condition resolved spontaneously without treatment and the mare became pregnant at this oestrus. (b) Moderate volume of uterine fluid in dioestrous mare. This fluid has persisted into the luteal phase and was associated with premature lysis of the corpora lutea and early return to oestrus. (c) Large volume uterine fluid accumulation in a mare with pyometra. This was treated by repeated catheterisation, lavage and administration of uterine antibiotics. The condition resolved and the mare conceived. (d) Moderate volume of uterine fluid in a mare with a long standing pyometra. There is increased echogenicity of the uterine wall (probably the result of marked fibrosis or calcification), the mare had cervical stenosis, and the pyometra was refractory to treatment.

(1) Infection which persists into the luteal phase, i.e. in the susceptible mare, becomes more aggressive because circulating progesterone further reduces the resistance of the endometrium thus allowing enhanced bacterial multiplication.
(2) Bacterial endometritis appears to stimulate premature production of uterine prostaglandin.
(3) This causes early regression of the CL (as soon as 7 days after ovulation).
(4) The consequent reduction in progesterone removes the inhibition on the uterine defence process, and allows the cervix to relax so that exudate can drain out.

NB: This condition is not easy to diagnose but should be suspected if:

(1) the mare has a discharge during interoestrus
(2) the mare returns to oestrus before 16 days or has a short interovulatory period (i.e. less than 19 days)
(3) the mare has palpable dilations in the uterus, a history of previous infection, or fluid in the uterine lumen when examined by ultrasound
(4) the mare has a muco-purulent discharge 7–8 days after parturition.

See Chapter 15 for treatment.

13.3 PYOMETRA

This term is usually reserved for situations where chronically accumulated pus causes marked uterine distention; however, ultrasound examination can identify small pockets of pus which can confuse the definition.

- Pyometra is not common in the mare because endometritis usually causes luteolysis with consequent relaxation of the cervix and drainage of the exudate.
- The development of pyometra usually requires two lesions:
  (1) endometritis
  (2) cervical abnormality (fibrosis or adhesions) which prevents drainage; however, some cases of pyometra associated with a normal cervix have been described.
- Diagnosis of pyometra is usually by rectal palpation of a large, thick walled, distended uterus; this can be difficult to differentiate from pregnancy without the use of ultrasound.
- Ultrasound examination will reveal a fluid filled uterus in the absence of a fetus. Ovarian findings may vary. The uterine fluid may be anechoic, or may have fine moderately echogenic particles, or large particles representing debris. The echogenicity of the fluid has little significance or relationship to the nature of the fluid.
- The mare may have a slight intermittent vulval discharge (associated

with times when the cervix is trying to relax, i.e. oestrus); this occurs when the cervix is slightly patent.

- Oestrous cycles may be:

  (1) short to normal in length; in this case luteolysis is usually being caused by premature prostaglandin release from the uterus
  (2) long; this is rare and occurs in chronic cases where the uterus is so damaged that it can no longer release prostaglandin and therefore the CL persists.

- Treatment is difficult but mainly relies on:

  (1) Induction of luteolysis with prostaglandin; this may cause sufficient cervical relaxation to allow some drainage to occur.
  (2) Attempting to catheterise the stenosed cervix and drainage of the uterus, by suction or siphonage.
  (3) Lavage of the uterus with large volumes of physiological saline at body temperature.
  (4) Three or four daily treatments (drainage and antibiotics) may be necessary, between each of which the uterus will involute further. Antibiotic treatment of the uterus should be carried out for 5 days after complete drainage.
  (5) Induce luteolysis as soon as possible after the next ovulation.
  (6) Attempts may be made to resolve cervical lesions, but most mares with pyometra have very poor breeding prospects and the condition often recurs if the mare is mated again.

13.4 VENEREAL BACTERIA (also see 16.2, 16.3)

The organism of contagious equine metritis (CEMO), also called *Taylorella equigenitalis* (formerly *Haemophilus equigenitalis*) and some strains of *Klebsiella pneumoniae* and *Pseudomonas aeruginosa* are considered to be venereal pathogens.

- Isolation of *Taylorella equigenitalia* is diagnostic since this bacterium causes contagious equine metritis.
- Not all *Klebsiella pneumoniae* are pathological; however, *Klebsiella* can be capsule-typed. Only capsule types 1, 2 and 5 have been implicated as the venereal pathogens.
- Not all *Pseudomonas aeruginosa* are pathological; however, serotyping is difficult and there appears to be poor correlation between serotype and pathogenicity.
- When deposited in the uterus of normal mares these bacteria cause an active inflammation (i.e. in the absence of pneumovagina, reduced uterine resistance or cervical lesions).
- This endometritis is persistent and may last for more than one cycle before it eventually resolves.

- This causes infertility because:

  (1) luteolysis is premature, and the mare returns to heat repeatedly and usually early
  (2) the mare is a source of infection to the stallion, who transmits the organisms to other mares
  (3) handlers and Veterinary Surgeons may also transmit the disease to other mares and stallions.

- Some mares, which may or may not have shown signs of previous endometritis, act as carriers of these venereal organisms.
- They harbour the organisms in the vestibular area, particularly the clitoral fossa and sinuses.
- Although they show no signs of infection, but they are potentially dangerous because:

  (1) mating or gynaecological examination may carry the organisms forward into the uterus, causing endometritis
  (2) the stallion may transmit these bacteria to other mares.

- It is interesting to note that:

  (1) stallions may harbour the organisms all over the penis (including the urethral fossa) and in the distal urethra, but show no signs of disease
  (2) CEM does not cause abortion, and mares have been known to discharge infected exudate from the vulva but have normal foals; the source of the discharge has not been ascertained
  (3) both sexes of foals from mares harbouring CEM in the distal genital tract can acquire the organism in their own genital areas. The mode of transmission is unknown as the foal is born in the intact amnion and doesn't contact the mare's genital tract during normal parturition.

NB: CEM is now a notifiable disease.

14 Swabbing and Biopsy Techniques, and Diagnosis of Endometritis

Swabbing of the mare's genital tract is carried out either to identify unaffected carriers of venereal pathogens, i.e. clitoral swabs (and penile swabs in stallions) or to diagnose uterine infection by cytological and cultural techniques.

14.1 CLITORAL SWABBING (FOR VENEREAL DISEASE CARRIERS)

- In Thoroughbreds the regulations for clitoral swabbing are described in the code of practice for controlling CEM (Appendix).
- Mares from which CEMO, *Klebsiella* spp. or *Pseudomonas* spp. are isolated should not be mated until they have been treated and reswabbed negative; however, only capsule types 1, 2 and 5 of *Klebsiella* and some strains of *Pseudomonas* are pathogenic and the course of action taken depends on the policy of the stud.
- Before taking the swab the mare should be adequately restrained (**3.1**) and standing in a position where her vulval area is well illuminated.
- Ideally an assistant should hold the tail to one side; if more than one mare is to be swabbed, the assistant should wear a separate disposable glove/sleeve for each mare.
- If faeces have caused gross contamination of the vulva, wipe with a dry paper towel but do not otherwise cleanse the area.
- The Veterinary Surgeon should also wear a sleeve on the hand used to evert the ventral vulva and expose the clitoris.
- A small swab (Fig. 14.1); is used to swab both the clitoral fossa and the central clitoral sinus (Fig. 14.2); in high risk mares, as defined in the code of practice, two swabs should be used, one for each site.
- Venereal pathogens live in smegma so that collection of this material from the sinus or fossa is advantageous.
- Clitoral swabs are immediately placed in Amies transport medium and sent to an approved laboratory to arrive during the working week.
- If the swab is moistened, sterile water should be used and *not* saline.
- Clitoral swabs are often not taken properly because:

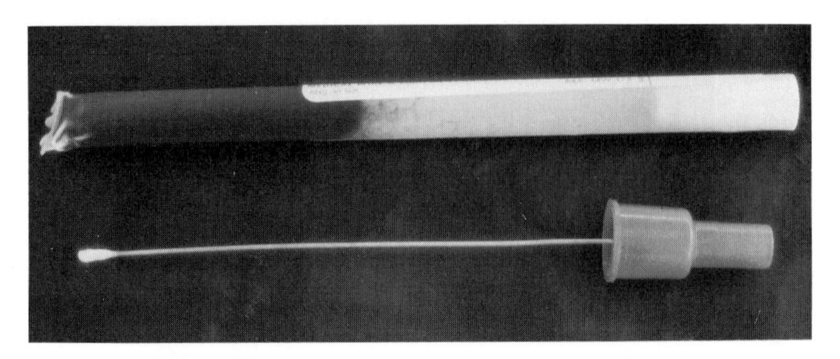

Fig. 14.1. A swab (and tube of transport medium) suitable for penetrating the clitoral sinuses.

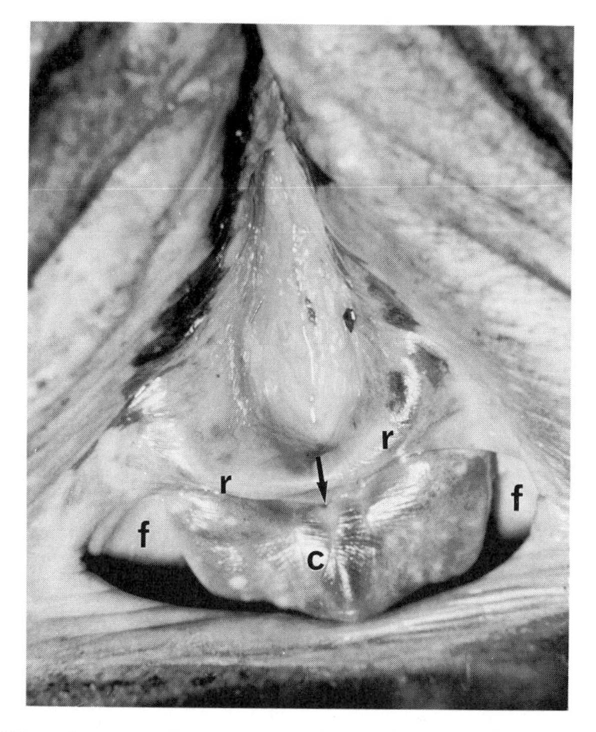

Fig. 14.2. Clitoral area of the mare: **c**, clitoris; **f**, clitoral fossa; **r**, clitoral frenulum; the arrow points to the opening of the central clitoral sinus.

(1) the swabs may be taken before the mare goes to the stud, in order to save time at the stud, by practitioners who are not conversant with the technique
(2) inadequate assistance makes proper swabbing very difficult, e.g. if no one is available to hold the tail

(3) penetration of the clitoral sinus usually evokes a pain-stimulated response from the mare; this may be dangerous to the operator and poor restraint can therefore prevent proper swabbing
(4) large swab tips may not penetrate the clitoral sinus
(5) failure to preserve the swab in the correct transport medium and to immediately dispatch it to the laboratory necessitate reswabbing.

14.2 UTERINE SWABBING

- Collection of material from the uterus is an essential aid for the diagnosis of endometritis.
- However,

  (1) approximately 30% of normal mares have some uterine bacteria
  (2) in some mares with endometritis, bacteria are not isolated from the uterus
  (3) the technique of swabbing may introduce bacteria into a previously normal uterus.

- Mares may be swabbed before mating to ensure that the uterus is not inflamed, and to check further for venereal and other pathogens.
- The common organisms isolated from mares with non-specific endometritis are β-haemolytic streptococci (BHS) and *Escherichia coli*; over 90% of infections are caused by one or both of these organisms. Occasionally α-haemolytic streptococci, non-haemolytic streptococci, staphylococci and *Proteus vulgaris* are found in mixed infections with BHS and *E. coli*.
- These organisms, along with many others, are normal inhabitants of the vulva and vestibular area, and only colonise the uterus for the reasons previously described.
- An ideal swabbing technique should therefore ensure that:

  (1) the swab enters the uterine lumen
  (2) the swab collects bacteria from nowhere other than the uterine lumen
  (3) the technique can be carried out with minimal assistance.

- Intrauterine swabbing techniques are of two types, i.e. via a speculum or using a manual, guarded swab.
- The former approach is most common in the UK and involves dilating the vagina and visualising the cervix with a vaginal speculum.
- Swabs are conventionally collected during oestrus, although there is an argument for collecting dioestrus samples since at this time bacteria and polymorphonuclear leucocytes should definitely be absent.
- **Always ensure that the mare is non-pregnant before placing a swab through the cervix.**

Speculum examination (13.5)

- Ease of visualisation of the cervix with a speculum depends on the type of speculum used, the type of horse examined and the amount of assistance available.
- Speculae are of two basic types.

The metal speculum

The metal speculum, e.g. the duck-billed (Russian) speculum (Fig. 14.3a). This was commonly used until recently; the advantage of this speculum is that the anterior vagina can be fully dilated giving a good view of the cervix to allow passage of a swab into the cervical lumen. A disadvantage of this speculum is that it requires sterilisation between mares; this can be achieved by having a number of speculae on the stud and sterilising in boiling water; short-term chemical sterilisation is inadequate.

Also a separate light source is necessary for illumination of the anterior vagina; if this is introduced into the vagina it is prone to contamination and should be protected.

Tubular speculae

Tubular speculae are of two types:

1. The most commonly used is the plastic tube which separately houses a protected light source (Fig. 14.3b). The tube sleeve can be resterilised although it eventually becomes opaque.
2. Recently a cheap disposable cardboard tube, slightly longer than the plastic version, has become available (Fig. 14.3c); a separate light source is necessary when using this method (e.g. a pen torch); the tube is 'silvered' to aid illumination.

- Both types have the advantage of allowing sterile examination of mares, but the view down the speculum is limited by the narrowness of the tube; occlusion by the passage of a swab down the tube limits vision.

NB: All intrauterine swabbing techniques using a speculum are potentially inaccurate because:

- the cervix can become contaminated with bacteria carried forward from the vulval lips and vestibule on the speculum as thorough sterilisation of the vestibule is impossible; the swab will collect these transferred organisms during examination
- contamination of the swab by inadvertent movement of the mare can occur when adequate assistance is not available, e.g. to hold the tail and to steady the mare
- light sources are often unreliable and may flick on and off
- it may be difficult to ensure that a swab has been passed through the cervical canal and into the uterus; this is most easy during oestrus but

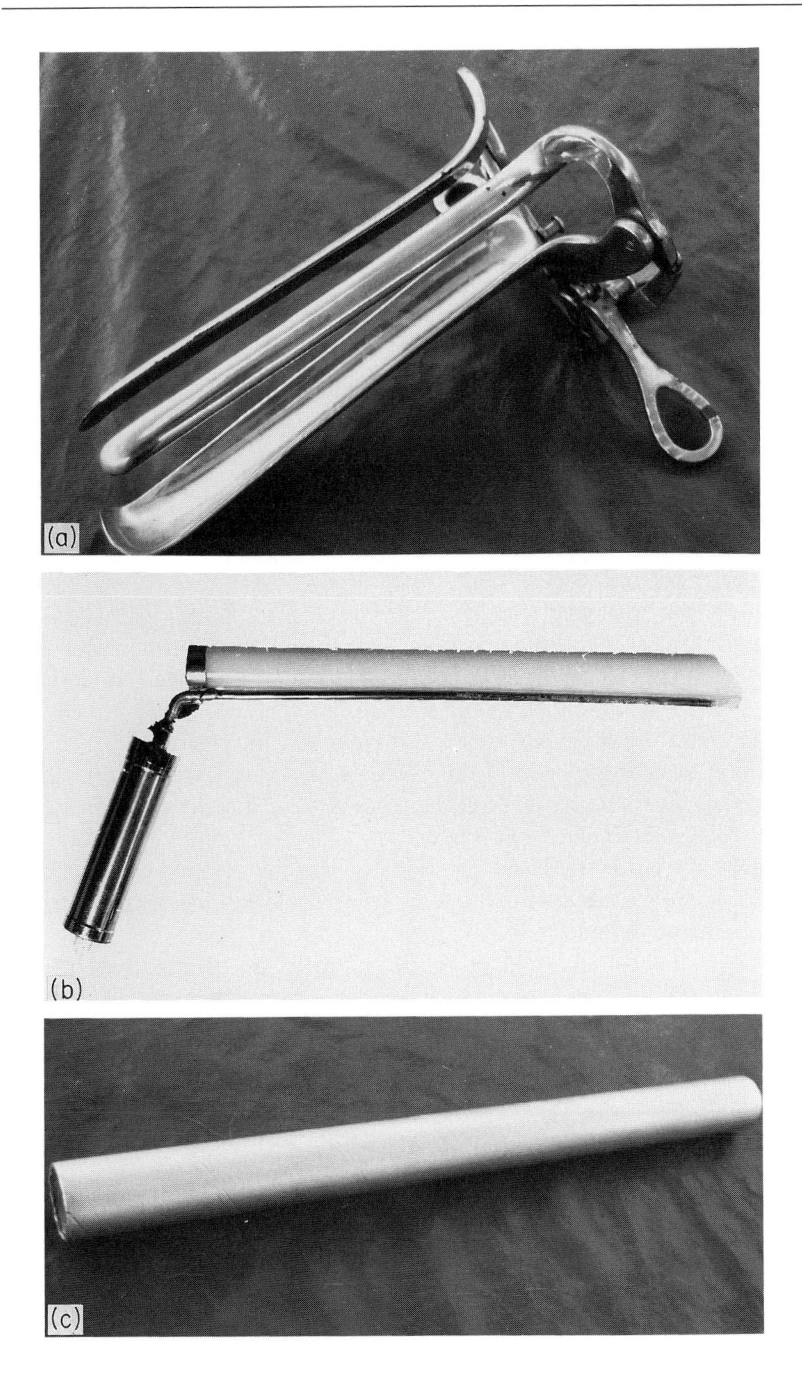

Fig. 14.3. Three types of vaginal speculum. (a) Metal (Polanski's) speculum. (b) Resterilisation plastic tube speculum with light source. (c) 'Silvered' disposable cardboard tube.

even then the canal may be convoluted and although patent may prevent easy passage of a swab

- in particular the precision with which uterine swabs can be taken depends heavily on the quality and quantity of lay assistance available – the average practitioner may only have one or two (inexperienced) helpers for this procedure, in which case less than optimal standards are inevitable.

Swabbing technique

- Whatever type of speculum is used, the vulva should be thoroughly cleaned beforehand and the tail covered with a disposable bandage or sleeve.
- Some authorities advocate the use of clean water and cleansing material to remove gross contamination (this helps to prevent bacterial resistance to antiseptics); others advocate use of various antiseptic substances.
- The speculum may be lubricated with an antiseptic-free gel (e.g. KY jelly) or warm water.
- Initially the speculum should be introduced through the vulval lips and pushed in a cranio-dorsal direction; after 5–10 cm a constriction (at the vestibulo-vaginal junction) is reached and further pressure is required to push the speculum past this.
- Thereafter the speculum is advanced cranially into the vagina.
- During oestrus the body of the cervix is positioned on the floor of the vagina and the external os is recognised as a spot or slit from which diverging oedematous folds radiate.
- Ideally the swab should be directed through the cervical canal without touching any other part of the tract, rotated a few times, and withdrawn in the same manner.
- If the vagina remains collapsed after insertion of the speculum (i.e. air does not enter the vagina) visualisation of the cervix is very difficult.

Guarded swabbing technique

- The alternative method of swabbing is to use a guarded technique; this has the advantage of being easy and accurate.
- The swab is housed in a plastic, metal or cardboard tube (the guard) which itself is housed in an outer tube.
- The operator uses a sterile sleeve, and places the swab along his/her dry, clean arm, inside the sleeve.
- The knuckles of the hand (sleeve) are lubricated with sterile jelly and the arm is inserted into the vagina, the cervix is located and the index finger is inserted against the os.
- The outer tube is advanced alongside this finger and finally pushed through the finger of the sleeve when further progression is impeded.
- Ideally the tube emerges from the sleeve at the tip of the index finger; in practice the point of penetration is usually within the cervical canal.

- Rupture of the sleeve should be sudden as very slow pressure stretches the sleeve excessively and may result in a thin film of plastic covering the end of the guard tube and subsequently masking the swab.
- Once the outer tube is within the cervical canal the guard tube is advanced.
- Once the guard tube has entered the uterus the swab is gently pushed out of the guard.
- When resistance is met the swab is rotated several times and withdrawn into the guard; the guard is then withdrawn into the outer tube. Excess forward pressure results in endometrial damage as the swab will contact the uterus immediately after it leaves the guard tube.
- The outer tube is now retracted into the sleeve and the arm withdrawn.
- The advantages of this method are:

  (1) no assistance is required, e.g. to hold the tail
  (2) the operator does not have to stand directly behind the mare
  (3) contamination is minimal
  (4) entry into the uterus is ensured.

- Disadvantages are:

  (1) the state of the cervix is not assessed visually
  (2) bacteria may be introduced into the uterus; these do not contaminate the swab and are eliminated rapidly by a normal mare in oestrus. However, problem mares, and those swabbed in the luteal phase may develop a subsequent endometritis. This may occur with any swabbing technique.

- Remember that breach of the cervix in pregnant mares will almost invariably cause pregnancy loss.

14.3 PROCESSING THE SWAB

Uterine (endometrial) swabs may be used for cytological examination and bacteriological culture.

Cytological examination

- If this is to be carried out it is best done by immediately rolling the swab gently onto a dry sterile slide; the swab can then be used for bacteriology.
- The smear may then be air, heat or chemically fixed depending on facilities; swabs which are placed in transport medium and used later for smears may have lost cellular material. Alternatively two swabs may be taken (the second is used for cytology).
- Various methods of staining are available – Leishman's, modified Wright–Giemsa ('Diff Quik'), methylene blue and Gram's are simple and

adequate; pre-stained slides are also useful (the main purpose of staining the smear is to show up polymorphonuclear leucocytes (PMNs). Trichrome stains are more complicated and take longer to perform.

- The smear is examined for (Fig. 14.4):

  (1) neutrophils (PMNs); these are not present in swabs from the normal uterine lumen and indicate inflammation
  (2) eosinophils which are occasionally seen in endometritis
  (3) endometrial epithelial cells which indicate that the swab entered the uterus or contacted exudate from the uterus; squamous epithelial cells come from the cervix and vagina.

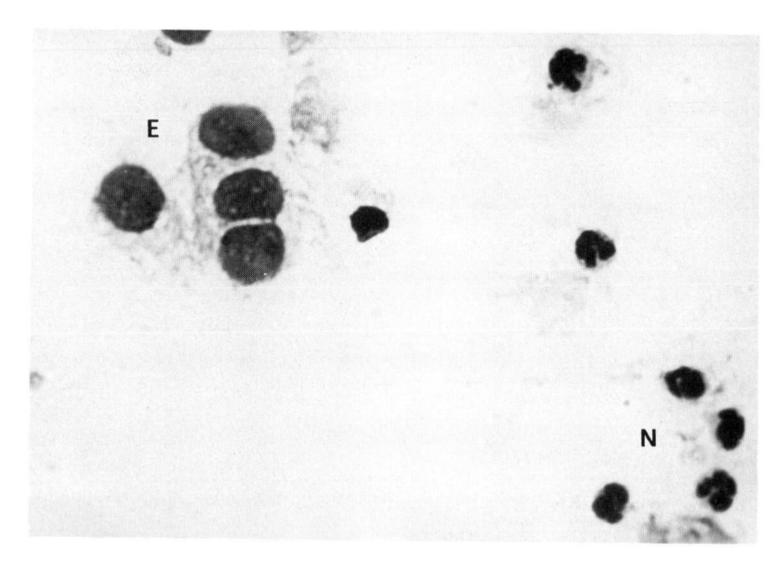

Fig. 14.4. Cells in a smear from uterine swab: E, epithelial cells; N, neutrophils.

Bacteriological culture

- All swabs should be placed in Amies' transport medium unless they are to be cultured immediately; this is essential when culture is for CEMO and desirable for all swabs; swabs which have dried in transit are useless (staphylococci, diphtheroids and fungi survive mild desiccation).
- All swabs should be dispatched to the laboratory immediately; if this is by post the swabs ideally should not be taken just before the week-end.
- Clitoral swabs must always be placed in transport medium; if the swab needs moistening before use (also for penile swabs in stallions) sterile water and *not* saline should be used; dipping the swab in transport medium first is ideal.

14.4 ENDOMETRIAL BIOPSY

Collection of the biopsy sample

- Endometrial biopsies can be taken from mares at any time, except during pregnancy or when complete fibrosis of the cervix is present. Mid dioestrus is a good time as it minimises misleading histological changes.
- Restrain the mare adequately (**3.1**), bandage the tail and cleanse and dry the vulva.
- Locate the cervix manually *per vaginam*, and dilate it with a finger; pass a sterile basket jawed forceps (Fig. 14.5) into the uterine lumen, and position this so that the cutting jaw faces dorsally.
- A biopsy of the dorsal body can then be taken 'blind' by lifting the open jaws of the forceps, closing quickly and giving a 'tug', or the uterus can be located *per rectum* and the jaws of the instrument guided to the junction of body and horn.
- Considerable traction may be required to sever the biopsy, as the instrument does not cut cleanly.
- Contrary to initial fears:

  (1) it is virtually impossible to rupture the uterus
  (2) haemorrhage is rarely significant
  (3) the mare appears not to feel the procedure.

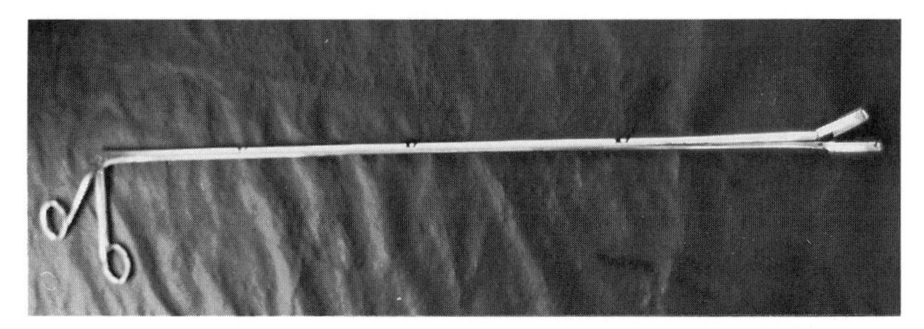

Fig. 14.5. Basket-jawed uterine biopsy instrument.

Processing the sample

- Remove the tissue from the basket gently with a hypodermic needle.
- Immerse immediately in buffered formal saline or Bouin's fixative; the latter penetrates the tissue rapidly but the specimen should be removed in 2–4 hours.
- Sections may be stained with haematoxylin and eosin, or more specialised stains, e.g. van Giesen for fibrous tissue.

Interpreting the biopsy

- Endometrial biopsies are useful as a diagnostic and to some degree as a prognostic aid. Accurate interpretation requires experience.
- Physiological changes include:

  (1) oestrus – tall ciliated epithelial cells and active glands which may contain secretions, and may be separated by interstitial oedema; glandular branches have a large diameter and are straight
  (2) dioestrus – low cuboidal epithelium with small inactive glands; glandular branches are often tortuous
  (3) anoestrus – inactive epithelium and sparce glands; this may be mistaken for atrophy.

- Pathological changes include:

  (1) acute inflammation – neutrophil and occasionally eosinophil infiltration
  (2) chronic infiltrative inflammation (probably due to repeated bouts of acute inflammation) – mononuclear cells (histiocytes, lymphocytes and plasma cells) in the stroma
  (3) chronic degenerative change – layers of fibrous tissue (lamellae) round 'nests' or dilated glands and diffuse stromal fibrosis; may also get dilated lymphatic lacunae. These changes are often associated with ageing
  (4) atrophy, hypoplasia, hyperplasia, tumours, etc.

  NB: Mares with chronic endometrial change may still conceive.

- A four category classification system has been proposed as a prognostic indicator of fertility:

  (1) Category I: normal endometrium. Greater than 70% of these mares will foal.
  (2) Category IIA: mild endometrial changes. Between 50 and 70% of these mares will foal.
  (3) Category IIb: moderate endometrial changes. Between 20 and 50% of the mares will foal.
  (4) Category III: severe endometrial changes. None of these mares usually foal.

- Prognosis is worse for older mares or mares which have been barren for two or more years.

15 Treatment and Prevention of Endometritis

15.1 GENERAL CONSIDERATIONS

- A normal transient endometritis occurs after mating and often after foaling; this is due to bacterial contamination, but post-coital endometritis may also be a reaction to seminal proteins and spermatozoa.
- It is considered that endometritis is usually caused by bacteria or yeasts and antibiotic therapy is therefore used.
- Lavage of the uterus with relatively large volumes of physiological saline may also have beneficial effects, since this will reduce the bacterial population, dilute toxic metabolites and remove cellular debris.
- However, methods of treatment are many and varied because the relative merits of intrauterine versus other routes of antibiotic treatment have not been extensively investigated (if i.m. or i.v. therapy is adopted, general recommendations for dose and length of treatment should be adopted).
- If intrauterine therapy is used, several aspects should be considered but there is no universally accepted method of treatment; the various criteria to be considered are:

  (1) which antibiotic should be used; usually there is insufficient time for the results of a sensitivity test to be acted on. However, the most common pathogens are β-haemolytic streptococci, *E. coli*, staphylococci and anaerobes (*Bacteroides fragilis*); antibiotics of choice are therefore penicillin, streptomycin, neomycin, framomycin, and nitrofurantoin (for anaerobes)
  (2) what volumes of agent should be infused; traditionally the antibiotic is suspended in large (100–500 ml) volumes of water or saline on the assumption that this volume is optimal for filling the uterus; however, the chemical effect of such dilution on antibiotic efficacy is unknown, and present evidence suggests that most of the antibiotic introduced in this manner is expelled through the cervix soon after treatment. The use of small volumes of antibiotic is appropriate on the assumption that the uterine lumen is only a potential space and therefore easily filled, and little of the agent is thereafter refluxed.

Also, if the antibiotic is absorbed from the uterus it should theoretically return to this organ again in therapeutic concentrations in the blood for some time after treatment
(3) the length of intrauterine treatment; this is governed by the stage of the cycle
(4) what stage of the cycle is best for the treatment of endometritis.

- If a mare has no history of chronic endometritis, and is not suffering from pneumovagina, there is little theoretical reason why she should have a positive uterine culture in early oestrus; however, these mares do occur, and consideration should be given to the possibility that contamination of the swab has occurred (in this case cytological investigation is valuable).
- Treatment may then be considered necessary at this stage, before the mare is mated, but since there is no evidence that endometritis is detrimental for sperm transport to the uterine tubes it is probably not necessary to withhold mating.

15.2 ACUTE ENDOMETRITIS

The most common indication for treatment or prevention of endometritis is in the mare which cannot cope with infection introduced at coitus. As previously discussed (**13.2**) this may be diagnosed by the detection of uterine fluid with ultrasound, cervical or vulval discharge, or uterine cytological or bacteriological examination.

There are several methods which attempt to reduce the magnitude of the post-coital endometritis including:

- using artificial insemination (**24.1**). Semen can be extended in a diluent containing antibiotic, and introduced into the uterus in an aseptic manner. This method is now more commonly used in the UK despite the resistance by the Jockey Club and some breed societies
- the minimal contamination technique; known susceptible mares have a large volume (100–500 ml) of semen extender, containing antibiotic, infused into the uterus immediately before service
- washing the mare's vulva and stallion's penis with water before coitus to remove gross contamination – the use of antiseptics is contraindicated (**27.2**).

Another technique is to allow normal coitus and then to treat the mare for any resultant endometritis. For accurate diagnosis to allow prompt treatment the mare should be examined no later than 24 hours after mating. Several treatment options are available including:

- antibacterial treatment after mating; this is intended to allow the usual (if ineffective) inflammatory response to develop but to treat this so that the uterus is normal by the time the zygote enters it 5–6 days after ovulation.

Antibiotic may be instilled into the uterus for up to 3 days after ovulation. Treatment before ovulation may be wasted if a second mating becomes necessary
- uterine lavage after mating; the uterus may be lavaged with large volumes of physiological saline to reduce bacterial numbers, dilute toxins and remove cellular debris. This has no detrimental effect on the subsequent pregnancy
- promotion of uterine drainage using ecbolic agents; intravenous and intramuscular administration of oxytocin is now widely used to stimulate uterine contractions and to promote drainage
- promotion of uterine drainage by cervical dilation; manual dilation of the cervix may allow uterine fluid to drain more freely into the vagina
- augmentation of the uterine defence mechanism; this has been attempted using colostrum or plasma from mares. Until the cause of infection in these susceptible mares is known, the value of such therapy is speculative
- Promotion of uterine drainage and treatment by the use of indwelling uterine catheters; however, these need suturing to the vulval area to reduce the likelihood of catheter loss, which nevertheless can occur; faecal contamination of the catheter can cause ingress of infective material.

15.3 CHRONIC ENDOMETRITIS

In the majority of cases the treatment options for chronic endometritis are the same as those described for acute endometritis. In addition some workers have attempted to stimulate inflammation, with successful resolution of the endometritis. Methods that have been advocated include:

- chemical cautery, e.g. 1% Lugols Iodine, although this may cause adhesions of the endometrium and damage to the opening of the uterine tubes
- physical cautery, i.e. scraping the endometrium with a special instrument
- intrauterine dimethyl sulphoxide.

15.4 URO-VAGINA

Some mares, usually those that have pneumovagina (**13.2**), also pool urine in the cranial vagina. This may result in a vaginitis and cervicitis. Urine may enter the uterus and cause inflammation, or bacteria may enter via the diseased cervix, especially during oestrus when the cervix is relaxed. The primary predisposing factor is pneumovagina. Treatment is by:

- removing any vaginal urine before mating with a pipette

- treatment of the uterus after mating as for acute endometritis
- treatment of the cause of the pneumovagina
- surgical reconstruction or lengthening of the urethral opening (Walker & Vaughan 1980).

15.5 CYSTIC ENDOMETRITIS

Endometrial glandular and lymphatic cysts are common in mares over 14 years of age (**8.10**, **12.13**) and may:

- cause no problems and go undetected
- be big enough to be mistaken for an early pregnancy, especially when at the base of a uterine horn; however, the absence of uterine tone would be suspicious (**8.2**)
- be mistaken for a pregnancy by ultrasound scanning, but they may not be the right size and shape or they may have been recognised previously; after 22 days an embryo should be seen in a pregnancy (**8.6**)
- numerous cysts may either prevent maternal recognition, or reduce the placental area sufficiently to affect the growth of the foal (**18.5**).

Treatment

Cysts may be visualised using an endoscope (before mating) and ruptured using the biopsy facility of the instrument.

15.6 PYOMETRA IS RARE (13.3)

Pyometra is the chronic accumulation of pus causing marked uterine distension.

- Treatment consists of passage, if possible, of a catheter through the cervix and aspiration of pus (a vacuum pump is useful). The pus may be very viscous and a large diameter catheter is usually needed. Aspiration should be followed by lavage with a large volume of physiological saline. Clearance of the pus and/or saline may be aided by administration of oxytocin. Antibiotics should be placed into the uterine lumen and the procedure must be repeated daily.
- After no more pus accumulates, antibiotic treatment is continued for 5 days. A total volume of 20 litres of pus is not unusual.

15.7 POST-PARTUM METRITIS

Post-partum metritis is a very serious condition which occurs most often in mares with retained placenta and is particularly serious in heavy horses, when it should be regarded as an emergency (**22.9**).

- Attempts to accelerate placental separation should be used (**21.3**).
- If placental separation is not complete (part is retained in the non-pregnant horn) or if post-partum metritis is suspected, at least daily lavage of the uterus is indicated; warm sterile saline (1–2 litres) should be introduced into the uterus, and immediately drained by siphonage; retention of some fetal membranes makes this difficult by blocking the drainage tube. A broad spectrum antibiotic should then be infused into the uterus; this should be effective against *E. coli* which is invariably present.
- Treatment is repeated until the pus and placental debris in the uterine exudate have disappeared.
- Supportive therapy with antihistamines, non-steroidal anti-inflammatory drugs, and parenteral antibiotic is helpful. Other treatments for endotoxaemic shock should be considered.
- Despite all efforts some mares die due to toxaemia or irreversible laminitis and pedal-bone rotation.

15.8 PNEUMOVAGINA

The treatment of pneumovagina is surgical (**13.2**) but intrauterine antibiotic therapy may be used before the operation to help the mare resolve her endometritis. Treatment regimes are usually modified from those described for the treatment of acute endometritis.

15.9 LOCAL CLITORAL TREATMENT

After isolation of venereal pathogens (**13.4**) from the vulval and clitoral area these sites must be rendered free of these organisms before mating can begin.

- The area should be thoroughly washed with water containing detergent to remove smegma from the clitoral fossa and sinuses; these areas are then packed with any topical preparation (not containing corticosteroid) of an antibiotic based upon its sensitivity. In the case of *Pseudomonas* spp. infection a 1 per cent silver nitrate aerosol may be used.
- Treatment is carried out daily for 5 days.
- Reswabbing after treatment is necessary (Appendix) to ensure complete removal of the potential pathogen.

15.10 CLITORAL SINUSECTOMY

Because of the inherent difficulties of swabbing and treating the clitoral area comprehensively, some mares in the past have remained positive for CEM without having been re-mated.

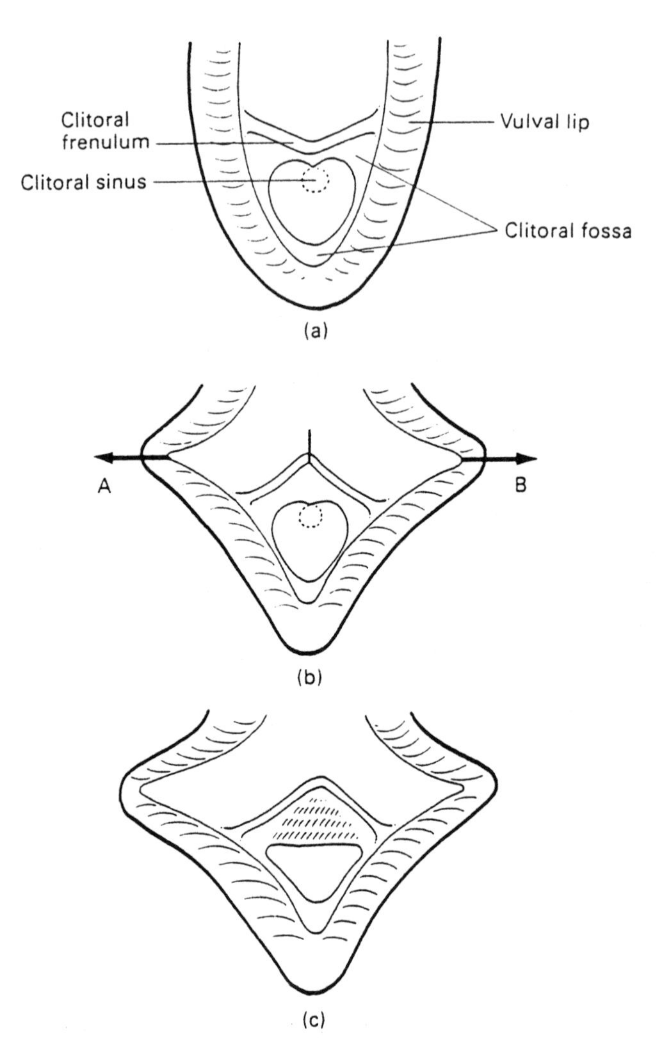

Fig. 15.1. Clitoral sinusectomy. (a) Restrain the mare, clean the vulva and note the anatomical sites. (b) Infiltrate the lateral vulval lips at A and B with local anaesthetic. These may then be retracted sideways using sutures, tissue forceps or retractors. Local anaesthetic infiltration into the clitoris and clitoral frenulum may not be necessary if the vulval block is adequate: retract the clitoral frenulum dorsally. (c) With rat-toothed forceps and curved scissors ablate the dorsal half of the clitoris, including the sinus; place this in transport medium for subsequent bacteriological investigation. Haemorrhage is usually minimal but may be staunched with an adrenalin-soaked swab.

- This led the authorities in North America to insist on removal of the dorsal part of the clitoris (including the sinuses) before mares could be imported.
- The operation involves local analgesia of the area, either by direct infiltration into the body of the clitoris, or local block in the vulval labiae; desensitisation of the clitoral frenulum is also necessary as this needs to be reflected dorsally to allow visualisation of the sinuses (Fig. 15.1).
- Excision of the dorsal clitoris should be such as to remove the central and lateral sinuses (if present) completely and the tissue is submitted for laboratory examination and culture.
- Subsequent haemorrhage is usually minimal, but USA and Canadian import regulations require follow-up local antibiotic treatment and swabbing, with supervision of the operation and post-operative treatment by an official from the Ministry of Agriculture.

16 Viral Causes of Infertility

16.1 EQUINE HERPESVIRUS 1 (EHV1)

EHV1 is the single most important cause of abortion in horses (the condition is discussed in **18.2**). It also causes respiratory (rhinopneumonitis) and nervous disease, and may cause significant disease in foals.

Important considerations are:

- EHV1 is *not* spread at coitus
- the predominant reproductive effects are abortion
- mares which have aborted are quickly free from the disease
- vaccination is available.

16.2 EQUINE HERPESVIRUS 3 (EHV3) – COITAL EXANTHEMA

EHV3 does not cause abortion in mares. Outbreaks are usually sporadic, and the initial cause is often difficult to determine.

- EHV3 *is* spread at coitus.
- Transmission may also be the result of veterinary examination with contaminated equipment.
- Mares develop vesicular lesions of the vestibule, vulval and perineal regions.
- Stallions develop similar lesions on the penis.
- Vesicles rupture and produce infected ulcers which usually heal well, although local antibiotic treatment may be necessary to resolve secondary infection.
- The condition usually resolves spontaneously within approximately 14 days.
- Fertility is only affected if the lesions on the mare or stallion are so inflamed that coitus cannot be achieved.

16.3 EQUINE VIRAL ARTERITIS (EVA)

EVA is a significant cause of abortion in some countries and there was an outbreak in the UK in 1993. The virus has a predilection for mucous membranes and other signs include conjunctivitis (pink eye), cough, dyspnoea, diarrhoea, colic, and subcutaneous oedema.

- EVA *is* spread at coitus (and also by chilled and frozen–thawed semen).
- EVA may be spread by droplet infection.
- The incidence of abortion is variable.
- Mares recover quickly from infection.
- Approximately 34% of stallions that are infected remain persistent viral shedders. These animals must be removed from the breeding programme.
- Recent work shows that whilst most Thoroughbred horses in the UK are seronegative, up to 50% of Standardbred horses are seropositive.
- Effective vaccination is available producing a low serological response.

17 Problems During Pregnancy

17.1 DEFINITIONS IN PREGNANCY DEVELOPMENT (see also 7.1–7.3)

Pregnancy failure is a term used to denote failure of a fertilised egg to develop into a foal born live at term. The consequences of such a failure depend largely on the stage of pregnancy at which death of the conceptus occurs. Various terms are used to describe the process of pregnancy development and pregnancy failure and its consequences; definitions of these terms are often not precise, but are best described as follows:

Embryo

This word is used to describe two entities:

- firstly after the fertilised egg (zygote) begins to divide, the resulting mass of cells is called an embryo
- at about 21 days after fertilisation this mass of dividing cells has differentiated into those which are going to develop into the membranes and umbilical cord, and those which are going to form the new individual. Once the potential individual separates itself from the surrounding membranes, it is called the embryo, or embryo proper.

Fetus

- The embryonic tissue which is destined to become a foal grows slowly initially, because the elements within it are moving and rearranging themselves.
- This primitive organisation of organ precursors is called organogenesis and the developing individual is known as an embryo until the process is complete (in the horse about 40 days).
- Thereafter the potential foal is called a fetus.

Conceptus

This is a blanket term and refers to all the products of conception throughout pregnancy, i.e. to the developing embryo or fetus plus its membranes and fluids, etc.

17.2 RESORPTION

The impression given by this word is that an established pregnancy is dissolved or digested and disappears with no trace.

- In fact, death of the embryo or fetus before about 4 months is usually followed by dehydration of the conceptus, i.e. all the fetal fluid (which constitutes the bulk of the conceptus) is resorbed into the mare's circulation, and the solid tissue (embryo/fetus and membranes) is dried out and degenerated due to autolysis (release of cell enzymes).
- The mare may not return to heat for some time. The products of resorption will be expelled, usually unnoticed, on return to heat.
- The stage of pregnancy at which fetal death is followed by immediate abortion, rather than resorption, is difficult to define as these events are rarely observed. Abortion of the conceptus is unusual before 40 days.

17.3 MUMMIFICATION

- Once a fetus has acquired a recognisable skeleton, i.e. after 4 months, continued presence of a dead fetus in the uterus results in the same dehydration process that is characteristic of resorption. However, in this case the bones will remain intact and the dehydrated fetus, a mummy, remains recognisable.
- This situation only occurs in mares in which one of twins has died, because death of a single foal causes abortion, unless the fetus becomes lodged in the cervix.
- Mummification therefore depends upon persistence of the corpus luteum.

17.4 ABORTION

Abortion means the expulsion of uterine contents before term. However:

- the dehydrated remnants of early pregnancy failure are likely to be voided unobserved
- fetal death is followed by abortion once the placenta has become responsible for progesterone production (**7.4**)
- abortion may occur in mares at grass and not be recognised because mares usually show no after effects of abortion, and predators soon scavenge the abortus and membranes
- abortion depends upon absence or loss of the corpus luteum
- because pregnancy length is so unpredictable in the mare, the stage at which premature expulsion of a fetus changes to normal term parturition is difficult to define, and subsequent description of events may depend on clinical assessment of the foal's ability to survive

- stillbirth usually refers to a dead foal produced after 320 years.

NB: All aborted fetuses or foals born dead or dying should be sent for expert post-mortem examination, especially where other in-contact mares are at risk.

17.5 PSEUDOPREGNANCY

This word is used to describe the reproductive phenomena which occur in the mare after pregnancy failure between 15 and 120 days of gestation.

- Pseudopregnancy type I occurs when the embryo dies before day 36.
- Pseudopregnancy type II occurs when fetal death occurs after day 36, i.e. during eCG (PMSG) production (**7.4**).
- The clinical features of these conditions will be described later.

17.6 PREGNANCY FAILURE

This subject is best considered by itemising events in chronological order. In general fertilisation rates are thought to be in excess of 90%.

Failure between 1 and 5 days

- Undoubtedly some fertilised eggs fail to develop further and die in the uterine tube.
- As is the case for unfertilised eggs, these never reach the uterus.
- The percentage of such failures is unknown.
- The mare has a normal oestrous cycle unless other events cause complications.

Failure between 5 and 15 days

- Fertilised eggs enter the uterus about 5 or 6 days after ovulation.
- Failure to develop further may be due to several causes, but those known are:
  - endometritis not only produces an environment (inflammation) unlikely to support pregnancy development, but also initiates premature lysis of the CL (**13.1**)
  - recent ultrasound studies have shown that some mares pregnant at 10–12 days are no longer pregnant at 17–18 days; this suggests failure of maternal recognition of pregnancy. The corpus luteum therefore regresses at the normal time or prematurely; cyclic oestrous behaviour is obviously resumed, usually at the normal interval, although mares may 'short-cycle'.

Failure between 15 and 36 days (Pseudopregnancy type I)

- If the mare has recognised that she is pregnant after 14–15 days the CL (corpus luteum verum) persists and the mare does not return to heat.
- Clinically, all the features associated with pregnancy develop in the tubular genitalia (**7.1**, **7.2**).
- Pregnancy failure results in resorption.
- Ultrasound imaging shows an initial reduction in volume of the conceptus (small size for age) followed by increased echogenicity of the fluids, inward bulging of the uterine wall, and finally loss of the normal appearance.
- Palpably the pregnancy bulge disappears due to dehydration, but:
  - all the other features of early pregnancy (closed cervix, tonic uterus, persistent CL, follicular growth) persist
  - the CL, which is responsible for those features (but cannot be palpated) may last for 2–4 months
  - this is pseudopregnancy type I.
- Natural demise of the CL, or its premature lysis by exogenous prostaglandin will cause rapid return to oestrus and expulsion of remnants of pregnancy (can this be called an abortion?).
- The induced heat should be as fertile as any other, but in practice it is less fertile particularly in pregnancies which have survived for more than 20 days.

Failure between 37 and 140 days (Pseudopregnancy type II)

- During this period eCG (PMSG) is normally produced.
- eCG complicates the endocrinological environment so that pregnancy failure during this period results in:
  - continued production of eCG until the endometrial cups regress naturally (there is no known method of accelerating their demise).
- The resulting syndrome is known as pseudopregnancy type II.
- For as long as eCG is produced the mare will not get in foal again.
- Two patterns of reproductive behaviour have been described during pseudopregnancy type II:

  (1) In ponies and some Thoroughbreds recurrent periods of oestrus occur with follicular development, but follicles become luteinised (i.e. produce progesterone) without ovulating.
  (2) In some Thoroughbreds the ovaries become small and quiescent and the mare enters a period of anoestrus.

Failure from 140 days to term

- The time when this period begins and the previous one ends is very variable because of the individual differences in the length of time that eCG remains in the circulation (60–200 days).

- Fetal death after eCG disappears from the blood is characterised by abortion because:
  (1) hormonal control of pregnancy at this stage is exercised by the fetus and placenta
  (2) fetal death is followed by a rapid drop in circulating oestrogen and cessation of progesterone production
  (3) these changes cause cervical dilation and myometrial contractions which ensure expulsion of the fetus and usually also the membranes.
- Because of the ease of abortion, mares rarely show signs of malaise and often abort unnoticed.
- After abortion the mare will come back into heat quite rapidly if this occurs in summer or spring, or may go into winter anoestrus if the pregnancy fails in autumn or winter.
- Fertility after abortion should be good, but:
  (1) retained placenta may be more common than after normal birth
  (2) bacterial cause of abortion may leave residual infection which requires resolution before conception can occur
  (3) abortion of twins may delay subsequent conception, presumably because of overdistention of both uterine horns.
- Rarely, possibly because of cervical stenosis, abortion is incomplete and fetal maceration occurs.

Premature and dysmature

Foals born before 320 days of gestation are arbitrarily defined as premature, although many of these survive; foals born after 320 days are sometimes weak and appear unprepared for extrauterine life; these are said to be dysmature.

In some mares apparently fully mature foals are born at approximately 320 days. Pregnancy length is variable and is shorter for foals born in summer and for pony mares (**7.8**).

18 Causes of Pregnancy Failure

18.1 BACTERIAL INFECTION

The presence of bacteria in the uterus after fertilisation prevents pregnancy development as previously described (**13.1**).

- It is unlikely that bacteria which enter the uterus at this early phase can persist and cause pregnancy failure later on.
- The organisms which most commonly prevent early pregnancy establishment are β-haemolytic streptococci and coliforms.
- These organisms and many others including *Aspergillus* spp. have been implicated in late abortion.
- In the latter half of pregnancy bacteria, yeasts and other fungi may enter the uterus via the vagina.
- A major cause of bacterial colonisation of the vagina is the mare developing pneumovagina due to loss of weight with subsequent vulval distortion (**13.2**).
- Bacteria which have entered the vagina cause inflammation, which eventually spreads forward to the uterus.
- Entry of bacteria into the uterus causes:

Localised placentitis (placental inflammation)

- If transient does not spread or endanger the life of the fetus.
- Evidence of such an episode is seen at term when the allantochorion around the cervix is noticed to be devoid of villi and is either thinned, or thickened with calcium deposits; there are histological signs of inflammation.
- Affected pregnancies may be prolonged due to impaired placental function and reduced fetal nutrition.

Extensive placentitis

- Affects sufficient placental area to seriously retard the development of the fetus, resulting in eventual abortion.
- Placental lesions are obvious and the aborted fetus may be small for its gestational length.

Bacteraemia or septicaemia

- Entry of organisms into the uterus via the mare's blood stream, or more commonly via the cervix, can result in immediate transferral to the fetus, with bacteraemia or septicaemia causing fetal death and abortion.

18.2 EQUINE HERPESVIRUS 1 (EHV1)

Equine herpesvirus 1 (EHV1) or rhinopneumonitis virus causes abortion in mares (especially sub type 1).

- The virus also causes respiratory disease; this is most noticeable in horses (foals and yearlings) which meet the virus for the first time.
- It may also cause paresis with ataxia, tail flaccidity and urine dribbling, or a fatal paralysis.
- Clinical signs of EHV1 infection of the respiratory tract are not distinguishable from those caused by other viruses (and secondary bacterial infection), i.e. nasal discharge, transient pyrexia and physical depression.
- Animals which have previously met EHV1 may become temporarily viraemic without showing clinical signs (usually older animals).
- The sources of the virus are:

  (1) clinically affected animals; nasal secretions contain virus in animals which are both obviously infected and those which fail to show clinical signs
  (2) aborted fetuses and their membranes
  (3) infected foals which are born live at term but which shed virus for the first week of life
  (4) mares which have aborted; these shed virus from the genital tract for only a short period, and can be mated after one month
  (5) unsuspected virus shedders.

- The epidemiology of the disease is complicated by latency:

  (1) after viraemia, virus can remain dormant (latent) in the reticuloendothelial cells of clinically normal animals for an unspecified length of time
  (2) activation of virus may be caused by stress or other factors
  (3) in pregnant mares this results in shedding and viraemia in the foal with subsequent abortion.

Diagnosis of EHV1 infection

- There is no test to detect latent carriers.
- Viraemia is followed by a short lived rise in circulating complement fixing antibodies (70 days); serum neutralising antibody remains elevated for longer.

- Virus isolation can be carried out on nasal secretions and fetal tissue.
- Post-mortem examination of aborted fetuses usually reveals marked peritoneal and pleural fluid and necrotic foci in the liver; lesions are also found in the spleen, adrenal glands and thymus.
- Virus can be demonstrated in fetal lungs, liver and thymus by fluorescent antibody test on snap-frozen tissue.
- These organs, particularly the liver, contain intranuclear inclusion bodies.

Epidemiology of EHV1

- Foals and yearlings usually first contract the disease by contact with infected peers or adults suffering recrudescence after latency.
- Pregnant mares are usually infected by:

  (1) clinically infected youngsters
  (2) abortus of other mares
  (3) infected foals born at term which may excrete virus for up to 9 days and yet may appear normal
  (4) clinically normal excreters.

- It is not known whether:

  (1) a mare can be carrying virus at time of conception, and abort later
  (2) aborted mares go into a further period of latency, but clinical experience suggest this is not so.

- Mares which contract the virus during pregnancy will usually show no respiratory signs (due to anamnestic response); therefore the time at which aborting mares had contracted the virus is unknown, unless samples are available for serology.
- Abortions can occur as early as seven days after exposure to virus and are usually seen after five months of gestation.

Control of EHV1 infection (Appendix)

Hygiene

- Keep weaned foals and yearlings away from pregnant mares.
- It is impractical on large studs to keep pregnant mares singly, but groups should be as small as possible and isolated from each other; this still may not prevent infection.
- Aborted fetuses and membranes should be sent for post-mortem examination where economically feasible.
- All other products of abortion and contaminated bedding should be burned.
- Aborted mares should be isolated for at least 1 week with strict control of admission to the box and routine hygienic measures.

- Outside mares should not be allowed onto infected premises until at least 1 month after the last abortion.
- Similarly, resident animals should not be allowed to leave for at least 1 month after the last abortion.
- Loose-boxes should be steam-cleaned and disinfected after being vacated by an aborting mare.

Vaccination

- Two vaccines against EHV1 are currently available in the UK, one dead and one attenuated.
- Only the dead vaccine is licensed for use in abortion protection.
- Experimental evidence cases doubt on their efficacy, but experience in the USA shows that regular and frequent vaccination reduces the incidence of abortion, and in particular prevents abortion storms.
- Vaccination should be considered where the cost relates favourably to the potential value of the foals at risk.
- Vaccination frequency is under review but should be as stated by the manufacturer.
- Ideally all horses on a premises should be vaccinated.

18.3 EQUINE VIRAL ARTERITIS (EVA)

Equine viral arteritis causes abortion in mares, and until 1993 was not present in the UK. Presently EVA is a notifiable disease under the Equine Viral Arteritis Order 1995.

- EVA is venereally transmitted, as well as being transmitted via the respiratory tract.
- The virus causes a wide range of clinical signs other than abortion including conjunctivitis (pink eye), cough, dyspnoea, diarrhoea, colic, and subcutaneous oedema. In the stallion there may be scrotal and preputial oedema. The severity may vary from slight pyrexia with conjunctivitis to severe illness.
- The sources of the virus are:

  (1) clinically affected animals, both mares and stallions, via nasal secretions (droplet infection)
  (2) aborted fetuses and their membranes
  (3) genital tract secretions for up to three weeks after abortion
  (4) infected semen (including chilled and frozen–thawed semen).

- The majority of stallions are infective only for a short period of time.
- 34% of stallions remain persistent viral shedders.
- The epidemiology of the disease is complicated by:

  (1) both coital and respiratory tract routes of transmission
  (2) persistent virus shedding in the semen of some stallions.

Diagnosis of EVA infection

- Horses may have characteristic clinical signs.
- Virus may be isolated from nasal secretions, aborted material and semen.
- There may be rising antibody titres.

Control of EVA infection (Appendix)

- Because EVA is usually only excreted for three weeks, a quarantine period exceeding this time should be considered.
- Screening of stallions for carrier status (antibody titre) is essential.
- Screening of the antibody titres of mares should be considered.
- A killed EVA vaccine is available in the UK on the basis of an Animal Test Certificate.
- Animals should be demonstrated to be seronegative before vaccination, and should be screened post vaccination to demonstrate that vaccine response has occurred. This is especially important in animals that may be exported, since it is necessary to demonstrate that the antibody titre is the result of vaccination rather than field exposure.
- All stallions and teasers should be vaccinated.
- The Equine Viral Arteritis Order 1995 allows stallions which shed virus to mate only seropositive or vaccinated mares.

18.4 MULTIPLE CONCEPTUSES (OFTEN TWINS) (see also 7.7 and 20.1–20.3)

The mare's placenta is structurally simple, and requires occupation of the whole endometrial surface to provide adequate nourishment to the foal.

- Twin pregnancies pose a problem because two fetuses are trying to develop with a placental attachment area designed for one (where the membranes of the two pregnancies meet, there is no placenta).
- In early pregnancy there appears to be a mechanism for causing death of the smaller of twins in some cases; this reduces the scale of later problems.
- If twins persist as pregnancy advances, the nutritional requirement of the fetuses increases, fetal growth is limited by placental attachment area and there are three common outcomes:

  (1) One fetus becomes larger than the other, the smaller, emaciated fetus dies and usually both are aborted at 8–9 months of gestation. This is the most common outcome (80% of cases).
  (2) The fetuses are similar in size, go to term and two small weak sickly foals are delivered. These may die or have to be destroyed.
  (3) The size difference between the fetuses is large and the smaller fetus

dies early in the pregnancy and is mummified. The larger twin is normally born alive and is able to survive.

18.5 MISCELLANEOUS CAUSES OF ABORTION

When the cause of an abortion is not investigated, it is easy to implicate some previous event, e.g. thunderstorm, kick by another horse, change in management, excess exercise, vaccination, worming, etc. In most cases these are merely incidental events, but being able to apportion blame is an understandable desire for the disappointed mare owner. Running the mare with a gelding does not cause abortion unless the gelding is 'riggy' and continually mates with the mare (**28.3**).

Causes of abortion

Some causes of abortion are:

- twisting of the umbilical cord; when the cord is tightly wrapped around the trunk or a hind limb it is probable that the circulation may be impeded sufficiently to cause fetal death
  (1) twisting the cord 'on itself' may be the result of fetal distress during an abortion, or may directly cause fetal death over a long period
  (2) evidence of previous (non-fatal) umbilical torsion is often seen when the urachus (thin walled) is dilated due to accumulation of urine or the bladder is grossly distended
- fetal abnormalities, e.g. hydrocephalus, occasionally stimulate abortion
- chronic endometrial change reducing functional placental area sufficiently to cause fatal malnutrition of fetus
- development of excess fetal fluid is very rare and may either stimulate abortion or necessitate therapeutic termination of pregnancy
- iatrogenic abortion is rare; drugs which are known to upset pregnancies in other animals are unlikely to be used in sufficient quantities in mares in late pregnancy (e.g. oxytocin, prostaglandin, xylazine, etc.)
- severe malnutrition at 20–30 days may cause resorption.

19 Other Abnormal Events During Pregnancy

19.1 UTERINE TORSION

- This can occur at any time during late pregnancy but is most common close to term.
- The uterus twists about its long axis to between 90 and 360 degrees.
- The mare shows signs of moderate to severe colic.
- Diagnosis is by examination *per rectum*; if the twist is anti-clockwise the right broad ligament can be felt stretched to the left over the dorsal surface of the uterus and vice versa.
- The prognosis for the foal is poor because of interference to the blood supply to the uterus (due to compression of the major vessels).
- The prognosis for the mare depends on the speed of diagnosis and treatment.
- Treatment is correction of the torsion via laparotomy, usually under general anaesthesia. If this is carried out in late gestation the pregnant mare may abort, but some will foal normally at term.
- Reduction of the torsion close to term is best followed by Caesarean operation via the same laparotomy.

19.2 VENTRAL HERNIA

- Rupture of the abdominal musculature and prepubic tendon occurs mainly in Shire and heavy horses in late pregnancy.
- This is characterised by massive ventral swelling and oedema, abdominal pain and often recumbency.
- Prognosis is poor although live foals may be produced by assisted delivery after parturition induction (**9.7.**) or Caesarean operation (**23.5**).
- Traction is usually required at natural foaling since the mare is unable to produce effective abdominal contractions.

19.3 HYDROPS OF THE FETAL MEMBRANES

Excessive fetal fluid may develop within the fetal membranes, although this is rare, causing:

(1) hydrops amnion
(2) hydrops allantois.

- Hydrops allantois is the most common, and is usually seen after seven months of gestation.
- Clinical signs include swollen abdomen and laboured breathing.
- Abortion may occur.
- Abortion should be induced if it is not spontaneous. Drainage of fluid and manual extraction is most appropriate.
- The condition does not necessarily recur at the next pregnancy.

19.4 PSEUDOPREGNANCY (17.5)

- Early embryonic and fetal deaths result in physiological events which usually mimic continued pregnancy, i.e. pseudopregnancy.
- However, by the end of the fifth month after conception, the pseudo-pregnant mare becomes capable of having normal oestrus cycles.
- Some mares, thought to be pregnant, put on weight and appear to have maintained gestation until examination at, or after, expected term shows they are not pregnant.
- Weight increase in this case is due to over feeding (because of expected pregnancy); there is no physiological basis for 'pseudo-pregnancy' as there is in the bitch in late gestation.
- Mares (and fillies) may have mammary development and even lactate at any time during their reproductive lives; this may be associated with increased feeding, especially grass, or other unknown factors.
- Lactation in non-pregnant mares usually stops without treatment, but may be curtailed by testosterone administration.

19.5 PROLONGED GESTATION (see also 7.8)

Gestation may extend between 310 and 370 days. Most mares that do not foal at the normal time are healthy and the owner should be reassured that this is probably normal.

- Excessive lactation before parturition may be associated with poor colostrum quality. Preparation should be made to provide the foal with an alternative source.

20 Reducing Infertility Caused by Multiple Conceptuses (e.g. Twin Pregnancy)

The incidence of multiple ovulations is approximately 20% in the mare. Should all oocytes that are ovulated be fertilised there is a high chance of pregnancy failure (**18.4**).

20.1 PREVENTION OF TWIN CONCEPTION

1 Avoid mating mares with two follicles; then use prostaglandins to shorten the interval to the next oestrus.
BUT

- the mare may not be examined regularly enough for detection of two follicles
- the mare may produce two follicles again at the next heat (this is common)
- it may be too late in the breeding season to miss mating at this heat.
- Detection of two follicles may be difficult because:

  (1) two follicles close to each other may feel like one large follicle on palpation, but these can be easily recognised by ultrasound examination
  (2) a follicle deep in the ovary may not be detected by palpation but would be seen imaged by ultrasound examination
  (3) a second follicle, unsuspected by palpation or ultrasound, may develop and ovulate during early dioestrus; if the mare was mated close to the first ovulation by a stallion with good semen longevity a second pregnancy could occur.

2 Try to mate between two anticipated ovulations, on the assumption that the ovum released before mating is unlikely to be fertilised.
BUT

- mating within 12 hours of an ovulation can still result in a conception
- both ovulations may occur between successive examinations
- the mare may go out of season before she has been mated
- such timing requires regular repeated examinations.

20.2 DIAGNOSIS OF TWINS

Manual palpation

- Even under ideal conditions this can be no more than 50% accurate, as in about one-half of twin pregnancies both conceptuses are in the same uterine horn.
- When twin pregnancies are in the same horn, they produce a single swelling at its base; contrary to expectations, this swelling often feels no bigger than a single pregnancy of the same age.
- Twins which are located in separate horns (bicornual) are easier to detect as two distinct swellings.
  BUT
- pregnancy examination at 21 days may miss bicornual twins as the younger conceptus may not yet produce a palpable swelling
- bicornual twins may be more difficult to detect in the post-partum uterus, although this arrangement is less common than in barren or maiden mares.
- The latest time for identification of bicornual twins by palpation is about 60 days – after this the two swellings become confluent; however, if twin pregnancy is to be terminated to give the mare a second chance to conceive during the current breeding season, diagnosis should preferably be before day 30.

Ultrasound examination

- Ultrasound gives a much more accurate diagnosis of twins than palpation, as the contents of the uterus are visualised (Fig. 20.1), but it is *not* 100%.
- At ultrasound examination the number of corpora lutea should be counted. Mares with two corpora lutea should be treated with suspicion (see **8.7** protocol for ultrasound examination).
- Examination for twins usually results in a reduced insurance premium on the life of the unborn foal.
- Twin pregnancies may be identified as early as 13–14 days (high frequency transducers are most accurate at this early stage).
- Wrong diagnoses may be caused by:

  (1) incomplete scanning of the uterus, which allows a twin to be missed
  (2) failure to recognise twins in the same horn because the plane of the ultrasound beam doesn't highlight the inter-conceptual wall; this can happen to the most experienced examiner, but is more common at 18–22 days before both embryos become visible, i.e. about day 25
  (3) endometrial cysts – these can easily be confused with pre-21 day pregnancies; regular repeated scanning is the only way to make the distinction accurately. It is preferable to have 'mapped' the shape, size and position of cysts before pregnancy diagnosis is required.

NB: After 60 days twin pregnancies are not diagnosable by palpation, and become rapidly more difficult by scanning.

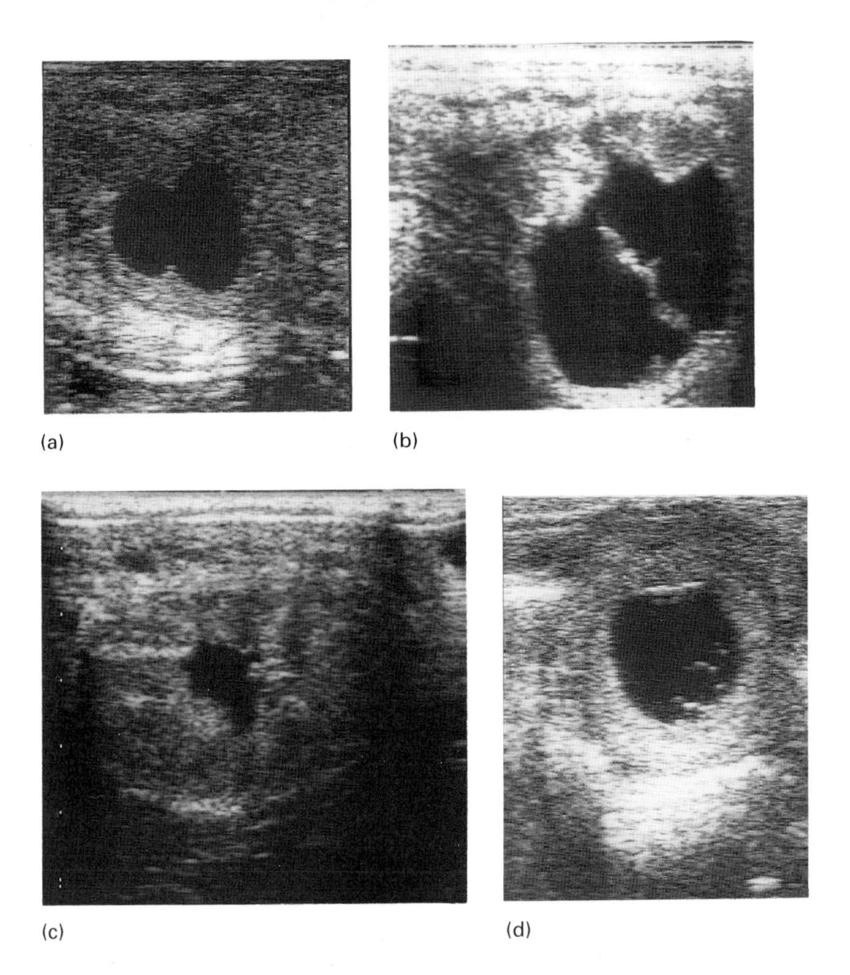

(a) (b) (c) (d)

Fig. 20.1. Ultrasound images of twin conceptuses (7.5 MHz transducer, scale in cm).
(a) 14 and 15 day conceptuses positioned adjacent to one another. At this time the conceptuses are mobile and can be separated. (b) 20 and 21 day conceptuses positioned adjacent to one another. At this time fixation has occurred and the conceptuses cannot be separated (the embryo can be seen positioned at the ventral pole of the lower conceptus). (c) Free uterine fluid after crushing of a conceptus. (d) Haemorrhage into a conceptus after repeated squeezing; this conceptus had disappeared when the mare was examined 24 hours later.

20.3 DEALING WITH TWIN CONCEPTION

- Some twin conceptions result in the birth of a single healthy foal, i.e. 'nature' ensures that one pregnancy fails early enough to prevent interference with development of the other.
- Differential growth rates can be identified using ultrasound.
- Frequently the conceptus which is small for its gestational age is the one that fails.
- Resorption is more likely for conceptuses that fix within the same uterine horn.

Coping with the problem

The clinician's dilemma is to decide whether and when to intervene. The decision must be made before day 33 if the mare is to stand a chance of getting in foal again during the same breeding season.

Interference with a twin pregnancy can be by:

- abolition of the whole pregnancy by lysing the corpora lutea with prostaglandin. If initiated before day 36 the mare will usually have a normal subsequent heat with average fertility; attempts to do this after day 36 (when endometrial cups secrete eCG) may not succeed and are unlikely to be followed by a fertile heat (**17.5**). It appears that in some mares endometrial cups are formed even when prostaglandin is given on day 32. In this case oestruses are usually associated with follicular luteinisation rather than ovulation.
- Manual rupture of one conceptus (Fig. 20.1(c)).

  (1) The smaller conceptus should always be chosen.
  (2) Early conceptuses (14–17 days) are not difficult to crush but as they are mobile in the uterine lumen they cannot always be easily fixed.
  (3) As the conceptus develops from day 21 greater pressure is required to rupture it, and after day 25, repeated attempts may be required.
  (4) As pregnancy proceeds after day 21, manual disruption of one pregnancy is more likely to be followed by death of the other, i.e. complete pregnancy failure. The reason for this is not known but it may be related to the larger volume of conceptual fluid that is released.
  (5) Bicornual pregnancies are most easily treated by this method, although gentle squeezing of two conceptions at the same site (unicornual) may be attempted in the hope that only one conceptus will be destroyed.
  (6) In some cases it may not be possible to burst one conceptus; however, repeatedly squeezing it may cause sufficient damage that it subsequently resorbs (Fig. 20.1(d)).

Assessing results

- Successful twin management usually requires early and repeated examinations.
- The initial ultrasound examination should be performed on day 14 or 15.
- Manual examinations after diagnosis and treatment of twins can confirm or otherwise the continuance of pregnancy.
- Ultrasound examination is superior, in the hands of an experienced clinician, as the course of development of twins or a surviving singleton can be monitored more accurately.

21 Retained Placenta

21.1 NORMAL EXPULSION

- The physical contact between the allantochorion and the endometrium is relatively weak, so that placental separation occurs rapidly after expulsion of the foal.
- Passage of the fetal membranes (cleansings, after-birth) is usually complete by three hours post-partum.
- However, it is traditional to consider that a problem exists if the mare has not cleansed by six hours after birth – all of these definitions are arbitrary.
- After a normal birth the membranes which are hanging from the vulva are the amnion (inner membrane) in which the foal was born, and the enclosed umbilical cord; the amnion may contain pockets of fluid (**7.3**).
- The weight of the amnion and cord result in the allantochorion separating from the endometrium at the point where the cord is attached to the allantochorion, i.e. at the base of the horn in which the conceptus first developed.
- Progressive traction by the amnion causes complete separation of the allantochorion, which becomes everted during the process (Fig. 9.1) and is passed inside-out.

21.2 EXAMINATION OF THE MEMBRANES

- Always check that the expelled membranes are complete.
- The amnion is usually torn but cannot be retained *per se*. It is a grey–white opaque membrane containing large blood vessels.
- Sometimes the amnion (and intra-amniotic umbilical cord) feels rough due to small plaques of epithelial cells; the significance of these is unknown but they are considered to be normal.
- The umbilical cord is usually twisted but not discoloured.
- The allantoic portion of the cord contains four thick walled vessels (two arteries and two veins).
- At the level of the attachment of the amnion, the two veins join so that only three vessels traverse the amniotic cavity to the umbilicus.

- Abnormal twisting of the cord on itself (**18.5**) or around a fetal limb etc. may cause distortion or haemorrhage into surrounding tissue.
- Sacculations are sometimes seen in the amniotic cord – these are dilations in the urachus and probably reflect short periods of mild twisting.
- The allantochorion should be spread out to ensure that all is present; its shape conforms exactly to that of the recently vacated uterus, i.e. a body and two horns.
- The outer surface is velvet-like due to villi and it is red in colour; differing intensities of colour occur normally due to hypostatic congestion with blood which was not expelled through the umbilical cord.
- The tips of the horns are avillous over a small ($\frac{1}{4}$ cm diameter) area where the chorion was against the uterine openings of the Fallopian tubes.
- The tips of the horns (especially the larger one) may be smooth and thickened due to oedema; the cause is unknown but this is thought to be normal.
- A haphazard arrangement of avillous areas, roughly forming a circle around the attachment of the umbilical cord, marks the position in the uterus of the now disappeared endometrial cups; there is also a small avillous area which coincides with the base of the cord – this marks the embryonic yolk-sac (bilaminar omphalapleur) placenta.
- The internal (non-placental) surface of the allantochorion is shiny and contains a mass of recognisable blood vessels.
- In a circular area round the attachment of the cord, and corresponding to the avillous area described previously, are little sacs on thin stalks (the chorio-allantoic pouches); these contain dead endometrial cup tissue and are normal.
- If a portion of the allantochorion is left behind it is invariably half or one-third of the smaller (non-pregnant) horn.
- Often the horns (and less commonly the body) are torn and it may be difficult to decide whether some membrane is missing and has been left inside or not.

21.3 ABNORMAL EXPULSION

- Immediately after the mare has foaled, the amnion hangs from the vulva to the level of the hocks or below.
- This may cause the mare to kick back, thus endangering the foal, or may be trodden on causing abnormal tension with a result that the membranes may tear, or the uterus may prolapse.
- To prevent this the membranes should be folded in two and tied without exciting the mare, to a position above the hocks.
- Baler twine is ideal for this, although the procedure is difficult due to the very slippery nature of the membranes.
- *Never* cut the amnion and cord off, as they provide the normal traction to produce natural separation of the allantochorion – also the amnion will retract back into the vagina taking bacteria and dirt with it.

- *Never* attach weights to the amnion and cord or pull on them; excess traction may cause rupture of the membranes or uterine prolapse (**22.7**).
- Retention of the membranes for more than six hours is often considered pathological because this sometimes results in metritis and laminitis, with fatal results.
- These severe sequelae are most likely in heavy horses following dystocia, following induced parturition, or in older mares, but are rarer in the lighter breeds (including Thoroughbreds) and ponies.
- However, because the literature is explicit as to these possibilities (because most of it was first written at a time when heavy working horses comprised the major part of the equine population), it is prudent to treat the condition as potentially serious.
- Most mares suffer few after effects in the presence of prolonged retention, whereas some heavy mares succumb to fatal sequelae even after prompt and thorough treatment.
- All mares with retained placenta should be visited.
- Ensure that the mare is adequately restrained in full view of the foal, which should be protected should the mare move violently around the box.
- Bandage the tail and cleanse the vulva as well as possible (the emergent membranes make this difficult). Well washed arms are preferable to gloves as differentiation between the tissues involved may be difficult.
- At this stage some part of the separating allantochorion may be visible at the vulva or palpable in the vagina.
- When removing fetal membranes manually, the reinforcement of the physiological method, i.e. tension via the umbilicus, cannot be exploited as traction may cause ripping of the membranes.
- If pieces of membrane are left in the uterus they are usually impossible to reach due to the disproportionate size of the recently evacuated uterus compared with the clinician's arm.
- Separation of the allantochorion from the endometrium is therefore attempted from the cervical end of its attachment (Fig. 21.1).
- The torn (cervical) end of the CAM is grasped (this contains the umbilical cord and maybe some amnion) and gently pulled caudally. The ends may lie well inside the vulva.
- Usually there is enough 'give' for this then to be held by a second hand at the vulva.
- At this stage the held allantochorion is twisted; this ensures that the force transmitted through the membranes is equally distributed throughout its attachment, i.e. that pieces of membrane are not pulled off piecemeal.
- With the allantochorion under tension, the hand in the tract is inserted between the CAM and endometrium and moved in a circular manner to separate the two.
- If separation is easy, i.e. the two components part like 'velcro' and there is no haemorrhage, then continued traction and tension on the exposed

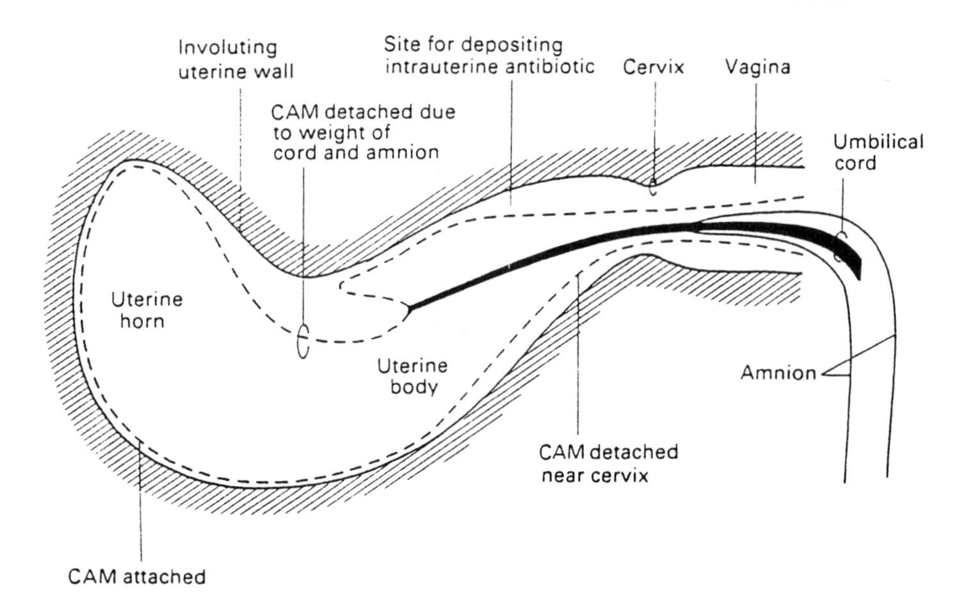

Fig. 21.1. Arrangement of the fetal membranes immediately after delivery of the foal (CAM, chorio-allantoic membrane).

CAM will bring the more anterior portions of the uterus into reach for similar treatment.

- Manual removal must be carried out with patience; the extent of success is difficult to determine – often the complete placenta separates when least expected.
- *However*, if manual removal is difficult, takes more than 10 minutes or causes haemorrhage, other treatments should be considered.
- Firstly, antibiotic may be infused into the uterus (see later), antihistamines or non-steroidal anti-inflammatory drugs given parenterally, and the mare revisited in 6–12 hours; several subsequent visits may be necessary before removal is complete.
- Secondly, oxytocin may be administered; some clinicians prefer this treatment as an initial approach.
- Ideally, an intravenous drip is established and 10–20 IU oxytocin given in 1 litre of saline over a period of one hour.
- The uterine contractions thus stimulated will hasten placental separation and may result in less micro-villous necrotic material being left *in utero*.
- This may be difficult if the mare is restless and is trying to 'nuzzle her foal'.
- Single doses of oxytocin (up to 40 IU) may be given i.m. but these are less physiological and large doses may cause excessive straining and uterine prolapse.
- After a complicated cleansing, heavy mares should receive continued antibiotic and antihistamine treatment and daily uterine lavage.

- This consists of infusing 500 ml warm sterile saline, and siphoning out the dark detritis.
- In the absence of saline, clean tap water should be used. Delay in removal of this material may result in irreversible toxaemia/laminitis.
- Similar treatment should be considered for mares which have retained some of the fetal membranes.
- Treatments should continue daily until the siphoned material is clear – if the aspirated material becomes purulent the mare has developed endometritis.
- In the author's opinion, neat antibiotic at the parenteral dose should be inserted after any intrauterine post-partum interference.
- If the membranes have not been expelled the location of the antibiotic should be chosen carefully, i.e. it must be deposited between the CAM and the endometrium. This is because absorption through the now dead allantochorion is probably poor, and because the bacteria introduced by the examiner's arm are likely to be between the endometrium and the CAM (see Fig. 21.1).
- Mares which have been slow to cleanse are unlikely to conceive at the foal heat; if mating at this heat is seriously considered the mare should be examined *per rectum* and *per vaginam*, and preferably using ultrasound, beforehand to assess involution (**10.2**).

22 Other Post-partum Problems

22.1 VULVAL AND PERINEAL TRAUMA

- Bruising of the vagina, vestibule and vulva commonly occurs during parturition.
- Deeper damage is only recognised if the mare is examined *per vaginam*; swelling of the vulval lips and adjacent perineal tissue is often observed and usually resolves within a few days of parturition.
- Vulval and perineal tears may occur in any direction but usually result from:

  (1) ripping at any angle either spontaneously or as a result of previous vulval closure which has not been opened
  (2) tearing of a normal vulva due to a large foal.

- Suturing is usually necessary, and can be carried out without local anaesthetic if the mare has foaled within the previous few hours. In cases of severe bruising or oedema suturing should be delayed for several weeks to allow devitalised tissue to slough.

22.2 RECTO-VAGINAL FISTULA (23.3)

Occasionally the foal's foot penetrates through the vaginal roof into the caudal rectum and causes severance of the vaginal roof and the rectal floor. Thereafter relaxation of expulsive efforts may result in realignment of the fetal limb and subsequent normal birth:

- In this case the recto-vaginal lesion often heals to form a fistula which allows constant access of faecal material to the vagina.
- This can only be diagnosed by careful examination *per vaginam* unless faeces are seen exiting the vulva.
- Treatment is difficult but relies on careful dissection of the fistula *per vaginam* and repair of the vaginal roof by suturing – treatment may be as for perineal laceration.

22.3 PERINEAL LACERATION

Penetration of a foot into the rectum may be followed by continued straining and trauma, resulting in recto-vaginal severance to the perineum:

- Post-partum, a rip between anus and vulva is evident, with gross contamination of the vagina/vestibule with faeces.
- The immediate treatment is antibiosis and supportive medication including protection of the wound may be necessary.
- Surgical treatment is delayed until the wound has healed by second intention, and the extent of the operative problem can be assessed.
- Under general anaesthesia (or local epidural block) an attempt is made to repair the vaginal roof, thus providing a reconstructed rectal floor.
- Several attempts may be necessary before an adequate surgical repair is achieved (Walker & Vaughan 1980).
- Mating should be withheld until the next breeding season.
- The anus may never function properly due to an inadequate anal ring.

22.4 RUPTURES OF THE CERVIX AND VAGINA *per se*

- These are rare and may result in peritonitis or pelvic abscess, depending on the site.
- Cervical damage is serious because subsequent fibrosis or adhesions (**13.3**) may compromise function and predispose to pyometra.
- Surgical treatment of cervical lesions is difficult and the prognosis for future fertility is poor.

22.5 UTERINE RUPTURE

- This occurs occasionally due to continued contractions during either an apparently normal parturition or during dystocia.
- If the mare's abdominal viscera are eventrated, diagnosis is easy.
- Uterine rupture may result in rapid onset of peritonitis and death despite supportive treatment (antibiotics, fluids, etc.).
- Occasionally the sequence of uterine involution and membrane expulsion may be such that peritoneal contamination does not occur, but adhesions between the uterus and adjacent viscera may form.
- If initial diagnosis is easy, and surgical facilities are available, uterine repair may be successful via laparotomy.

22.6 HAEMATOMA

Rupture of the uterine vessels or their branches is not uncommon.

- Smaller vessels bleed into the space between the myometrium and its serosal covering until the build up of pressure produces haemostasis:
  (1) In this case the mare may exhibit mild signs of colic after delivery.
  (2) Examination sometime later will reveal a fluctuant or hard mass on the surface of the uterus.
  (3) Resolution of the haematoma occurs slowly, and usually does not affect the ability of the mare to conceive again.
- Extensive haemorrhage ruptures the uterine serosa. The mare shows moderate to severe signs of colic with progressive anaemia. Diagnosis is difficult (the immediate post-partum uterus cannot be palpated in its entirety) and the outcome is usually fatal.

22.7 UTERINE PROLAPSE

- This is uncommon in the mare and may occur immediately after expulsion or due to traction on fetal membranes or straining.
- It is probably more common after dystocia.
- The everted endometrium is very vascular and easily recognised.
- Fatal haemorrhage may occur if the uterus is traumatised.
- Epidural anaesthesia may be used but this often takes a long time to work and is usually unnecessary with adequate restraint of the mare.
- The membranes should be removed and the uterus carefully lavaged.
- Lifting the uterus helps to reduce congestion and facilitates replacement if help is available.
- The uterus is 'fed back' from the vulval attachment (vagina) using a clenched fist and copious lubrication.
- Replacement is usually easier than in the cow and should be followed by insertion of a clean bottle or large volumes of saline to ensure complete eversion of the horns (saline should subsequently be siphoned off).
- Suturing of the vulva is unnecessary, but may be requested by the owner.
- Supportive treatment involves antibiosis, antihistamines, non-steroidal anti-inflammatory agents and calcium; oxytocin is contraindicated as this stimulates further uterine contractions.
- In heavy horses, daily uterine lavage and antibiosis is indicated (**21.3**).
- Fatal toxaemia may occur despite treatment.

22.8 HYPOCALCAEMIA

- This is rare in the mare and usually occurs immediately pre- or post-partum.

- The condition is more related to stress than calcium metabolism *per se*, and characteristically occurs in feral horses which have been housed prior to foaling.
- Mild cases involve slight hyperaesthesia and very dry faeces. These are followed by inability to prehend foot (which worsens the condition) and the onset of diaphragmatic asynchrony ('thumps').
- Severe signs are recumbency accompanied by tetanic spasms.
- Treatment is the slow infusion of calcium borogluconate to effect with continuous monitoring of cardiac activity.

22.9 POST-PARTUM ENDOMETRITIS

This condition is dealt with in Chapter 15.

22.10 MANAGEMENT OF THE ENGORGED MAMMARY GLAND

This may occur either at planned or unanticipated weaning. In many cases treatment is not warranted.

- Restricting water, and feeding only hay, may reduce lactation.
- Milking and lavage of the udder only provide further stimulus for milk production and may initiate mastitis.
- The mare may be uncomfortable for 24–48 hours post-weaning, but non-interference with the udder is advisable.
- When mastitis does develop, stripping of the gland (every 2–4 hours) is initially beneficial, with appropriate systemic antibiosis.
- When the gland is no longer hot (despite the degree of induration), milking should stop; usually the lack of attention to the opposite gland has reduced the rate of milk production.
- Remember that although there are only two teats, there are four sections to the mammary gland each with a teat orifice.

23 Dystocia

23.1 DEFINITIONS

Dystocia

Any problem which interferes with the normal birth of the foal.

Presentation

The direction the foal is facing relative to the long axis of the mare; this can be:

- anterior longitudinal, i.e. normal – the foal's head is presented towards the mare's vulva (preceded by the feet); a late pregnancy examination may often confirm this presentation
- posterior longitudinal, i.e. the foal is 'back-to-front' and the rump is presented first, preceded by the feet (in most cases – see breech below)
- transverse – this implies that the foal lies at right angles to the mare's spine, i.e. it occupies both uterine horns. In reality the foal cannot lie transversely across the mare's abdomen and appears to be in a longitudinal presentation. Thus the uterus is distorted to accommodate this rare presentation.

Position

This describes the relationship between the foal's back and the mare's spine; normal birth is accomplished in the dorsal position, i.e. foal's back uppermost.

- During later pregnancy the foal may lie on its side (lateral position) or back (ventral position) but rotates during late first and early second stage parturition – this may fail to occur during induced parturition.

Posture

The disposition of the extremities (neck and limbs), relative to the body.

- Essentially these are either extended (as the neck and forelimbs are in normal birth) or flexed.
- Hip-flexion in posterior presentation results in 'breech birth'.

- Flexion of the forelimbs may be unilateral or bilateral and involve any joint, and may occur in normal limbs or those with tendon contractions.
- Head and neck flexion only occur in anterior presentation and may be associated with ankylosis (fusion) of the cervical vertebrae (wry-neck).
- Unilateral or bilateral flexion of the hind limbs, when the foal is in anterior presentation results in the so-called 'dog-sitting' position which may be impossible to diagnose by palpation *per vaginam*.

23.2 SIGNIFICANCE OF DYSTOCIA

- Despite the long limbs of foals, dystocia is uncommon in the mare.
- Luckily, the most severe forms of malpresentation are the rarest.
- Sadly, dystocia more often results in death of the foal and maybe the mare because:

    (1) the mare usually continues with expulsive efforts, even if the foal is 'stuck'
    (2) the placenta separates rapidly during labour and unless the foal can breathe it soon loses its oxygen supply and dies
    (3) continued unproductive straining by the mare may cause damage to her reproductive tract
    (4) uterine damage during dystocia can cause fatal peritonitis or haemorrhage
    (5) retained placenta, as a result of uterine inertia following dystocia, can be fatal
    (6) uterine prolapse may occur.

23.3 RECOGNITION OF DYSTOCIA

1 The foal is normally born in anterior presentation, dorsal position and extended (head, neck and forelimbs) posture.
2 Failure to observe the fluid filled amnion (which may be visible only during contractions) at the vulva after five minutes of second stage parturition indicates that vaginal examination is necessary and may reveal:

- Two feet (one anterior to the other) and a nose, i.e. normal birth – delay could be due to:

    (1) feto-maternal disproportion or fetal oversize. This is rare in mares except the smaller breeds of pony
    (2) hydrocephalus impeding passage of the enlarged head through the cervix. This is rare
    (3) slow relaxation of the cervix (for example after induction of parturition)

(4) ineffectual straining. This is rare
(5) dorsal deviation of one or both feet – if unrecognised and not corrected this can cause recto-vaginal trauma (**22.2**, **22.3**)
(6) slowness of the fetus to rotate into normal dorsal position – this is recognised by inability of the fetlocks to flex ventrally, but they will do so dorsally or laterally, and the limbs may be crossed.

- One foot and nose – carpal and/or shoulder flexion of one forelimb.
- Nose only – carpal and/or shoulder flexion of both forelimbs.
- Two limbs only; this could be:

(1) head and neck flexion – carpi flex in a ventral direction unless position is also wrong
(2) posterior presentation with hind limbs extended; these flex in a dorsal position and the hocks should be palpable – recognition of the tail will help diagnosis.

- Nothing palpable in the vagina – this is serious and indicates:

(1) transverse presentation – may recognise fetal abdomen in the uterus
(2) posterior presentation with bilateral hip flexion (breech)
(3) anterior presentation with bilateral limb and head/neck flexion.

- Tough allantochorion identified – no fluid loss identified and the vagina is still relatively dry. Foal being born in CAM and placenta separating. NB: This must be distinguished from an unopened cervix; often an owner will misinterpret discomfort and grunting for second stage labour.
- Very rarely, prolapse of the mare's bladder causes dystocia.

23.4 NON-SURGICAL TREATMENT OF DYSTOCIA

Restraint

- Most mares are too concerned with foaling to worry about manipulation *per vaginam*.
- However, due to discomfort the mare is disinclined to stand still.
- If the mare wants to lie down and roll, this can often be an advantage if it is proving difficult to manipulate the foal into a dorsal position.
- A bridle and/or twitch may be useful but should not be relied upon.
- Tranquillisers may make early manipulation easier, but will reduce straining when this could be helpful.
- Epidural anaesthesia has the same advantage and disadvantage as tranquillisers – additionally the response is slow and variable.
- Introduction of a stomach tube into the trachea prevents the mare from straining.
- Parenteral clenbuterol may help to stop mare straining.
- General anaesthesia may be considered for final manipulative attempts before a surgical approach.

Manipulation

- Whilst awaiting experienced help it is best to walk a mare with dystocia, to stop her from straining; this prevents further loss of fluid and reduces trauma to the reproductive tract.
- Vaginal examination should be made with a washed and lubricated ungloved hand – this aids the differentiation of the vaginal wall (if the cervix is closed), allantochorion and amnion.
- If the allantochorion is still intact it must be ruptured using a finger (nail), guarded knife or hypodermic needle – this membrane is very tough.
- If the amnion has not ruptured it is best to assess the situation, and carry out preliminary manipulations through the membrane; this prevents loss of amniotic fluid and facilitates repositioning of appendages.
- Initially attempts are made to ascertain the cause of dystocia and thereafter to correct abnormalities of posture and position – the latter involves the following techniques:

  (1) repelling any part of the fetus which is in the vagina, to allow access to flexed appendages
  (2) application of ropes to the head and fetlocks
  (3) application of blunt eye hooks
  (4) the introduction of warm water or saline into the uterus where all the natural fluids have been lost
  (5) applying traction to the foal, or attached ropes, once satisfactory posture and position have been achieved.

- Problems encountered during manipulation are:

  (1) observers often expect rapid results and do not understand the difficulties involved
  (2) the mare may be uncooperative
  (3) pain (due to the mare straining) and tiredness of the operator's arms make manipulation progressively more difficult
  (4) drying of the mare's vagina makes her resentful of repeated re-insertion of the arm – it is helpful to lubricate the arm regularly but not the operative hand (which is less effective when slippery)
  (5) the ruptured amnion, particularly when trying to apply ropes to the head, constantly insinuates itself between hand and foal, and prevents the rope from gripping
  (6) preventing a head (which appears reluctant to be born) from flopping back into the uterus can be difficult; this probably reflects failure of the body of the foal to rotate and it may be helpful if the mare is allowed to roll.

- Whilst applying traction to a foal, always consider:

  (1) Is the vagina adequately lubricated?
  (2) The direction of pull – once the fetal head is clear of the vulva the foal should be pulled towards the mare's hocks.

(3) The strategy of traction – try to ensure that limbs are pulled alternately and in unison with the mare's straining efforts – retain tension on the head.
(4) Could the fetus be oversized? This is rare.
(5) Have the hips locked? Once the head and forelimbs are delivered the rest of the birth should be easy. If this is not so it may be because of hip lock or hind limb flexion (dog-sitting position); the latter cannot be diagnosed. In this case repel the foal if possible and rotate it into a lateral position – a large rotation of the front of the foal probably only affects the hips to a minor degree – and pull again.

- When the foal is born by traction, the mare is often standing. Once the thorax starts to pass through the vulva call for assistance to support the foal to prevent trauma from falling and premature rupture of the cord (**9.5**).
- If the mare is recumbent after delivery pull the foal's forelegs round to the mare's head to establish contact.
- Allow the cord to rupture spontaneously; do not ligate it; if haemorrhage occurs apply a haemostat temporarily.
- After any delivery, particularly if it is easy, check for a second fetus.
- The time at which manipulation and/or traction will have been considered to fail will depend on many factors, not least the possibility of quick surgical intervention.

23.5 SURGICAL TREATMENT OF DYSTOCIA

Embryotomy

- Embryotomy involves the removal of part of the foal, *per vaginam*, either using a roughened wire or a knife.
- Embryotomy is best performed by an experienced obstetrician with appropriate guards to prevent trauma to the reproductive tract.
- Embryotomy should only be considered in the mare if it is felt that one incision will be sufficient to allow rapid delivery of the fetus or if there is no alternative.
- The most likely situations when embryotomy will be applicable to the mare are:

(1) hydrocephalus – removal of the head may be facilitated by first puncturing the cranium and releasing fluid
(2) irreducible head/neck flexion
(3) where there is no alternative.

- Consideration should always be given to the likelihood of vaginal/uterine trauma sustained by the mare.

Caesarean operation

- This operation is elected for in cases of irreducible dystocia, or when it is considered that prompt surgery may produce a live foal.

- Anaesthetic and surgical procedures always pose some risk to both dam and foal, and these should not be overlooked.
- The salient points of the operation are as follows:

  (1) The anaesthetic given to the mare should be one which causes minimal depression of the foal, e.g. induction with xylazine and ketamine and maintenance with halothane.
  (2) A pre-mammary gland mid-line approach is probably best.
  (3) On gaining entrance to the abdomen the uterus is immediately apparent; a recognisable part of a fetal appendage (usually a hock) should be located through the uterine wall and an incision should be made through a relatively avascular area.
  (4) An incision of about 23 cm will allow exteriorisation of first one limb (after digital rupture of the amnion) and then the other, but help will be needed to pull the foal clear of the abdomen.
  (5) If the foal is alive it should be held for a while, in a position which doesn't compromise the asepsis of the operation, to allow emptying of the placental vascular bed through the umbilicus; however, attempts to ensure that a potentially viable foal is breathing take precedence, and it is wise to clamp the umbilicus before severence.
  (6) Contamination of the abdomen with fetal fluid, especially after a prolonged dystocia, should be minimised, although this is not always possible. Large volume lavage of the peritoneum with physiological saline may be necessary if this occurs.
  (7) After clamping any vessels in the uterine wall which are bleeding, the allantochorion is identified and peeled back from the endometrium.
  NB: It may be difficult to distinguish the allantochorion from the endometrium – attempts to separate the endometrium from the myometrium will result in haemorrhage, which may be severe.
  (8) After separation of the allantochorion, the endometrium is opposed to the rest of the uterine wall, round the complete periphery of the incision, using a locking stitch.
  (9) The uterine wall is closed with a Lembert or Cushing suture, avoiding the allantochorion; if the latter membrane is included the uterus may be prolapsed during third stage parturition.
  (10) After closing the abdomen, the mare should be allowed to recover sufficiently for a natural bonding to occur when the foal is presented.
  (11) As well as antibiotic and fluid therapy if required, the mare should be given a small dose (5 IU) oxytocin i.v. to aid involution and expulsion of the membranes and fluids.
  (12) Post-operative complications include uterine and vaginal haemorrhage, shock, wound breakdown, herniation and laminitis.

24 Manipulation of Reproduction

24.1 ARTIFICIAL INSEMINATION (AI)

- The use of AI in the UK is increasing because the authorities, except Wetherbys, will now allow registration of foals born as a result of AI.
- The objections to AI by the Thoroughbred registration authorities are presumably because of the possibility of individual stallions being used to produce excessive numbers of foals, and because the system could be abused, with parentage subsequently being attributed to the wrong stallion; this latter objection is now eliminated by blood testing.

Advantages of AI

These are as follows:

- Insemination is easy in the mare; the insemination catheters can be passed into the uterus by manual guidance *per vaginam*, and if necessary the catheter can be directed *per rectum* into the uterine horn ipsilateral to the ovulating ovary.
- One ejaculate can be divided into several portions, especially if an accurate insemination technique is performed as just described.
- Busy stallions need only to be collected from once every two days under normal circumstances.
- More mares can be inseminated from a particular stallion than by normal service.
- Semen can be transported more easily than the stallion, for mares some distance away.
- Semen can be stored for use after the death of a stallion.
- Dilution of semen in extender containing antibiotic reduces the risk of venereal (and other) bacterial disease (**13.4**).
- Similar treatment to semen reduces uterine contamination for mares with poor uterine immunity (**13.2**).
- Regular collection of semen from stallions allows constant checking of seminal quality and bacterial content.

Disadvantages of AI

These are the following:

- Collection may be difficult, hazardous or impossible, especially if the stallion is not used to the procedure.
- A mare in season is necessary, preferably one that stands quietly, although stallions can be trained to jump dummies and some can be collected from without mounting.
- Theoretically a stallion could become overused in a particular mare population.
- Semen from some stallions is not suitable for chilling or freeze–thawing.
- Wilful deceit could result in a mare being inseminated with the wrong, or erroneously labelled semen; however, in the author's opinion this is no more likely or undetectable than mating a mare with the wrong stallion.
- Since collection and insemination are usually carried out by a Veterinary Surgeon, the cost would usually be increased.

Collection of semen

Semen is collected by:

1. An *artificial vagina (AV)*. These are costly but provide an environment similar to the normal vagina (**26.3**).

    - The stallion is allowed to mount a mare in heat, and his penis is directed into the AV.
    - Most stallions accept the AV but some are very reluctant to ejaculate into it.
    - The collector is well-advised to wear protective foot and headwear.

    NB: This is the method of choice.

2. *Rubber condoms or breeder's bags*. These are available in the USA, and are placed over the stallion's penis before he mates the mare; the condom is removed at dismount.
    Plastic 'rectal' sleeves are sometimes placed over the stallion's penis in a similar manner, but are liable to rupture.
3. *Dismount sample*. This is the fluid ejaculated by many stallions during withdrawal, especially if the penis is still erect.

    - If the stallion's penis goes flaccid whilst still in the mare's vagina, fluid often escapes from the vulva on withdrawal.
    - In either case it is composed mainly of viscous, seminal vesicle secretion.
    - If, however, adequate spermatozoa are present, insemination of this material into a mare might be worthwhile; the advantages of disease control are, however, negated.
    - Evaluation of such a sample only gives a rough guide to the quality of the ejaculate (**26.4**).

The use of artificial insemination

- Fresh (diluted) semen insemination may be used:
  (1) when there is inability to mate with the mare (aggressive mare, unwilling stallion, mare injury)
  (2) to reduce venereal pathogens
  (3) to inseminate more than one mare
  (4) for minimal contamination techniques used to control endometritis.
- Semen may be stored for a short period of time by chilling and rewarming:
  (1) this allows transportation of semen
  (2) it may be useful when there is short-term unavailability of the stallion.
- Semen may be stored for long periods of time by freezing and thawing:
  (1) this allows transportation of semen
  (2) genetic material may be stored for a long period of time.
- Several pathogens may be spread in equine semen:
  (1) EVA
  (2) CEMO
  (3) *Klebsiella* and *Pseudomonas* species.
- Legislation concerning artificial insemination:
  (1) breed authorities: may or may not permit AI within a breed
  (2) Ministry of Agriculture, Fisheries and Food: control of semen imported into UK
  (3) General Stud Book: regulates the Thoroughbred breed.

Semen preservation

- Semen may be preserved:
  (1) fresh and cooled to room temperature
  (2) diluted and cooled to 5°C
  (3) diluted and frozen (–196°C) then thawed.
- The lifespan of preserved semen depends upon the preservation method:
  (1) fresh semen: four hours (although this may be extended by initial dilution)
  (2) diluted and cooled semen: 48 hours
  (3) diluted and frozen semen: indefinite.
- Semen is normally diluted in an 'extender solution' which aims to:
  (1) protect spermatozoa during cooling/freezing/warming
  (2) supply an energy source to spermatozoa

(3) maintain pH, osmolarity and ionic strength.

- For many species the optimal pH for survival is approximately 7.0. During storage hydrogen ions are produced by spermatozoa; therefore the pH falls. Control of pH is important and many agents have been used:

  (1) phosphate buffer
  (2) egg yolk
  (3) milk proteins
  (4) zwitterionic buffers, e.g. Tris, Tes, Hepes.

- Hypotonic diluents are harmful since they lead to a gain in intracellular water and redistribution of ions. Hypertonic diluents are less harmful since they lead to water loss and a reduction in the likelihood of intracellular ice crystallisation. Seminal plasma is 300 mOsm; thus most diluents are approximately 370 mOsm.
- Glucose, fructose and mannose are glycolysable sugars that may be included in semen extenders as sources of energy.
- The larger molecular weight sugars (ribose, arabinose) are often used as non-penetrating cryoprotectants.
- Antibacterial agents are usually included in semen extenders to control proliferation of microorganisms including pathogenic venereal bacteria.
- Specific protective agents may be used including:

  (1) milk proteins which protect against cold shock
  (2) egg yolk (low density lipoproteins) and bovine serum albumen which protect acrosomal and mitochondrial membranes, and protect against cold shock.

- Cryoprotective agents are essential for semen freezing since they prevent ice crystal damage. Cryoprotectants may be divided into those that are:

  (1) penetrating (e.g. glycerol and DMSO)
  (2) non-penetrating (e.g. sugars and polyvinyl pyrollidone).

Preparation and use of fresh stallion semen

- Fresh semen can be inseminated immediately after collection.
- Care should be taken to avoid too rapid cooling of the semen (temperature shock).
- If semen is not required for a short period of time it may be stored at room temperature.
- If semen needs to be stored for more than 1 hour before use it is best diluted with an extender (it is common to use the extender described for chilled semen – see below).

Preparation and use of chilled stallion semen

- A common extender is composed of: non-fat dry milk (e.g. Marvel), 2.4 g; glucose, 4.9 g; sodium bicarbonate, 0.15 g; sufficient deionised water to make the volume up to 100 ml. Antimicrobial agents may then be added; penicillin 150 000 IU, and streptomycin 150 000 mg.
- The semen is collected, the gel fraction is removed and it is diluted with the extender at 37°C.
- The extended semen is cooled slowly to 5°C and stored at this temperature.
- Semen may then be transported before being inseminated.
- It is important to perform a trial storage before shipping semen.
- A simplified method is commercially available: the Hamilton–Thorn Equitainer System.

Preparation and use of frozen–thawed stallion semen

- Semen is collected and diluted with an extender containing sodium citrate, 3.7 g; glucose, 60.0 g; disodium EDTA, 3.7 g; sodium bicarbonate, 1.2 g; deionised water, 1000 ml.
- The diluted semen is centrifuged to form a sperm pellet.
- The seminal plasma is removed and the pellet is suspended in a second extender containing lactose solution (11%), 50 ml; glucose–EDTA solution, 25 ml; egg yolk, 20 ml; glycerol, 5 ml; penicillin/streptomycin as above.
- Samples are slowly cooled to 5°C and allowed to equilibrate for 2–4 hours.
- Samples are then loaded into 0.5, 1.0 or 4.0 ml straws (vials/plastic bags are also used).
- Straws are frozen at standard freezing rates in liquid nitrogen vapour, before being plunged into liquid nitrogen.
- Straws are generally thawed rapidly (70°C for 10 seconds) before being placed at 37°C.

Success with preserved semen

- Spermatozoal longevity is greatest for fresh diluted semen, and least for frozen–thawed semen.
- Fertility rates are related to spermatozoal damage during preservation and to spermatozoal longevity.
- Extensive mare management is required when frozen–thawed semen is used, since the timing of insemination has to be very close to the time of ovulation.
- It may be extremely difficult to preserve the semen from certain stallions; the reason for this is not known.

24.2 EMBRYO TRANSFER

Non-surgical embryo transfer is possible in the horse.

- The technique of embryo collection is relatively simple, i.e. the embryo is flushed out of the mare's uterus 7 or 8 days after ovulation.
  (1) This requires the infusion and subsequent collection of physiological solution, which is introduced through the cervix of the conscious mare in the standing position.
  (2) The embryo is quite easily identified and can be inseminated into the uterus of a mare at the same stage of the cycle, using a specially designed pipette which ensures delivery of the embryo.
  (3) Scrupulous asepsis is essential during ovum insertion to avoid bacterial inflammation-induced luteolysis.
- The advantages of embryo transfer are:
  (1) embryos may be collected from a valuable mare which is thought to be otherwise unable to maintain a normal pregnancy, e.g. due to age, uterine damage, prepubic tendon rupture, etc.
  (2) several embryos may be collected from one mare of an endangered breed during one breeding season, thus increasing the number of foals of that breed born the following year
  (3) the technique helps with the understanding of fundamental physiological aspects of equine reproduction, e.g. when donkey embryos are transferred to horse mares, etc.
- Problems with embryo transfer in the mare are as follows:
  (1) Superovulation is difficult to stimulate so usually there is only one embryo after each successful collection; research in this field may be fruitful in the near future.
  (2) Due to the long follicular phase of the mare's oestrous cycle, it is very difficult to synchronise ovulations (i.e. between donor and recipient); it is therefore usually necessary to have several potential recipient mares for each donor.
  (3) This makes embryo transfer expensive because of the number of mares which must be kept and monitored closely for each possible success.

24.3 MICROMANIPULATION OF EMBRYOS

- The use of genetic engineering has had little impact on horse reproduction to date.
- However, successful splitting of the mare egg, fertilised *in vitro*, with subsequent production of identical twins in two recipient mares has been reported.
- Further development in this field is likely.

25 The Normal Stallion

25.1 ANATOMY (Fig. 25.1)

The scrotum

- This is the sac which contains the testes. The scrotal skin is usually hairless (except in donkeys and small ponies) and shiny.
- The scrotum can change in shape to regulate the proximity of the testes to the body and thus help to control their temperature.

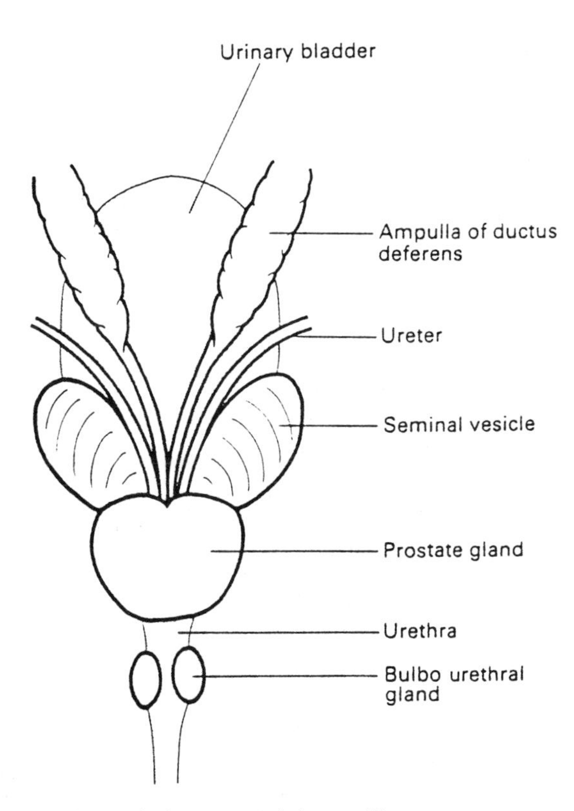

Fig. 25.1. Intrapelvic genital organs of the stallion.

- A septum divides the scrotum into two halves, one for each testis.
- The inner lining of the scrotum (tunica vaginalis communis, or parietal layer of the tunica), is separated from the testicular covering (tunica vaginalis propria or visceral layer of the tunica) by a thin film of fluid – this allows easy movement of the scrotal skin over the testis.

The testis (testicle)

- Those of a Thoroughbred stallion are about 10 cm × 6 cm × 5 cm; the size of the testis is roughly proportional to the size of the horse.
- Both testes are normally of a similar size with one lying slightly cranial to the other.
- Palpably the testis is firm, smooth and regular in shape.
- The testis lies with its long axis horizontal.
- There is some correlation between testicular size and spermatozoal production.

The epididymis

- A very long tube in which spermatozoa, which have left the testicle, mature.
- The tube is tightly coiled upon itself and the resulting oblong structure is attached to the testis.
- The head of the epididymis is on the cranio-dorsal pole of the testis.
- The body of the epididymis runs caudally on the dorso-lateral aspect of the testis to the
- tail, which can be palpated on the caudal pole of the testis and is about $2\frac{1}{2}\,cm^3$ in the Thoroughbred; equine spermatozoa are infertile until they enter the tail of the epididymis.

The spermatic cord

This is a complicated structure which contains:

- the spermatic artery
- the spermatic vein; this is spread out into a complex network of small veins (the pampiniform plexus) which surrounds the spermatic artery and cools the blood which is going to the testis
- the cremaster muscle which can (with the scrotal skin) vary the distance of the testis from the body wall and thus influence its temperature
- the ductus deferens (vas deferens).

The ductus deferens

- This tube is a continuation of the epididymis, and transports spermatozoa from the latter to the urethra.
- It enters the horse's abdomen (with the cremaster muscle, testicular vessels and their supporting tissues) through the inguinal canal.

- In the abdomen the ductus deferens becomes dilated to form an ampulla, in which spermatozoa are stored temporarily.

The inguinal canal

- This channel is formed by a gap in the abdominal muscle, just anterior to the scrotum.
- Soon after birth (usually within two weeks), the foal's testes should have descended through this canal and entered the scrotum; failure to do so results in a cryptorchid – if only one testis is undescended it is a unilateral cryptorchid; if both are undescended it is bilateral. The term monorchid refers to a horse with only testicle – this is extremely rare (**28.3**). Anorchidism, a congenital absence of testes, is also very rare.
- If the inguinal canal is too large, intestine may pass through it and cause an inguinal hernia (**27.3**); this can occur in colts or stallions or soon after castration.

The urethra

- This tube connects the opening of the urinary bladder to the tip of the penis, and conveys urine to the outside.
- It also transports semen during ejaculation.
- The intra-pelvic portion of the urethra is joined by three sets of glands:

  (1) the prostate which partially surrounds the urethra
  (2) a pair of large seminal vesicles which lie just on top of the bladder
  (3) a pair of smaller bulbo-urethral glands which are caudal to the seminal vesicles.

- In the penis, the urethra is covered by the bulbo-spongiosus muscle, whose contractions force semen and urine along the urethra.

The penis

- This is usually housed within the sheath and is composed mainly of two erectile tissues, the corpus spongiosum penis and corpus cavernosum penis.
- During erection the penis has a mechanism for filling with blood which cannot normally escape until after ejaculation.
- The stallion's penis is relatively long when erect, and slightly dilated at its distal tip.
- During ejaculation further swelling of the tip occurs – this dilates the mare's cervix and helps to ensure that most of the ejaculate enters the uterus; this extra swelling can be seen if the stallion dismounts from the mare before ejaculation is complete.
- At the tip of the penis the urethra opens through the tubular urethral process (Fig. 25.2); this process is surrounded by the urethral fossa (or fossa glandis), which dorsally adjoins a further dilation, the urethral diverticulum. These latter two cavities are sites of smegma accumulation.

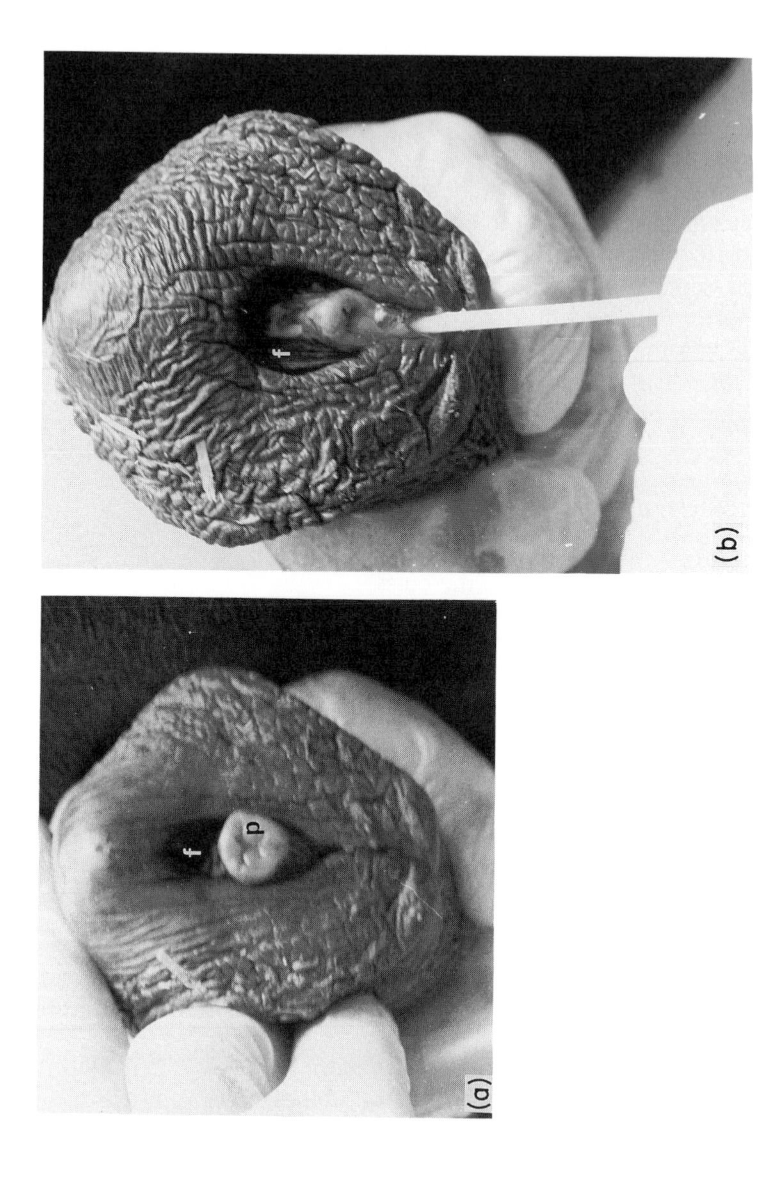

Fig. 25.2. (a) Tip of stallion's erect penis showing urethral process, **p**. (b) A swab is in the urethra; the urethral process is surrounded by the urethral fossa, **f**.

The prepuce or sheath

This is the structure in which the inactive penis is housed (Fig. 25.3).

- Laterally and ventrally it is composed of skin.
- Internally, in the resting state, it is doubled-back on itself forming the preputial fold; this fold straightens out during erection.
- Smegma also accumulates in this fold and at the base of the penis (**26.1**).

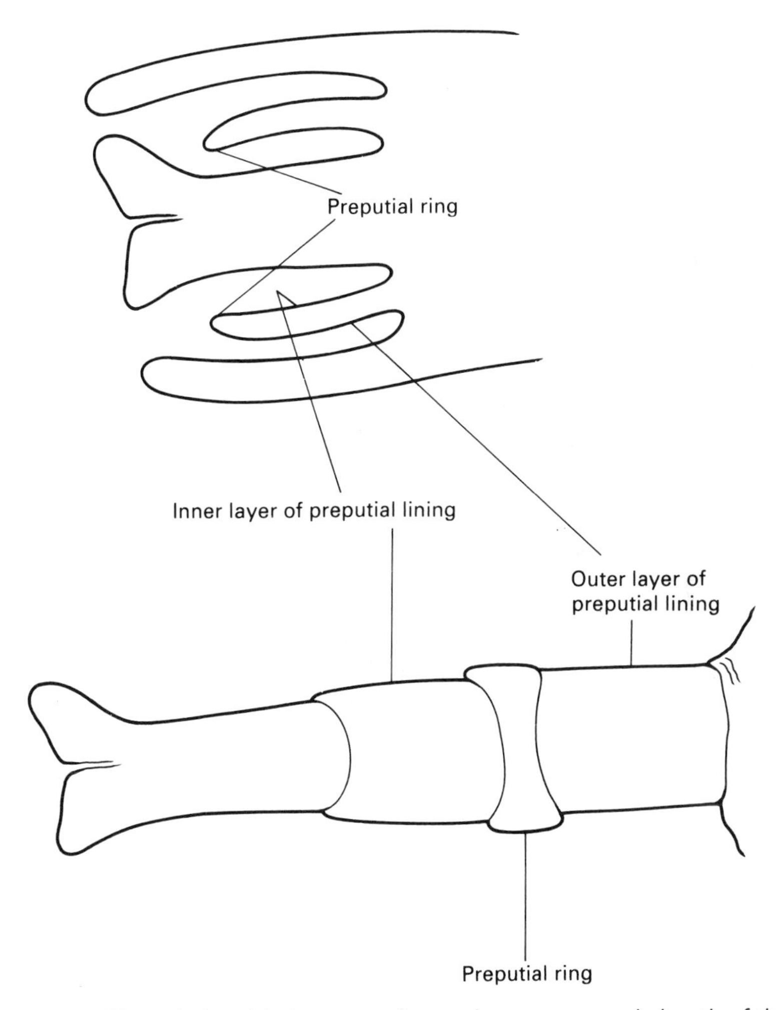

Fig. 25.3. The relationship between the penis, prepuce and sheath of the stallion.

25.2 ENDOCRINE CONTROL

Gonadotrophin release is regulated primarily by the episodic stimulation of the pituitary gland by gonadotrophin releasing hormone (GnRH).

- LH and FSH (to a lesser extent) are secreted into the peripheral circulation by the anterior pituitary gland in an episodic manner.
- The functional significance of this pulsatile release is not known.
- LH secretion is immediate but transitory after GnRH stimulation.
- FSH secretion is slow and gradual.
- The half life of FSH is also longer than that of LH. Therefore the plasma changes in LH are more rapid than those of FSH.
- LH binds to specific receptors on Leydig cells of the testis and stimulates testicular steroidogenesis.
- Testosterone secretion occurs both locally within the testis and into the peripheral circulation.
- Peripheral concentrations of testosterone are necessary for the development and maintenance of secondary sexual characteristics, maintenance of sexual behaviour, and negative feedback regulation of gonadotrophin secretion. The production of testosterone within the testis is important for initiating and maintaining spermatogenesis.
- High intratesticular testosterone concentrations are maintained within the seminiferous tubules, in part, by the binding of testosterone to androgen binding protein.
- FSH binds to specific receptors on the plasma membrane of Sertoli cells.
- Androgen binding protein is produced by the Sertoli cell under the influence of testosterone and FSH.
- FSH binding results in the production of a variety of proteins that are important in regulating spermatogenesis.
- Feedback control of FSH is via the gonadal peptide inhibin.
- Inhibin is a non-steroidal glycoprotein product of the Sertoli cell that selectively inhibits FSH secretion at the pituitary gland.
- Other negative feedback mechanisms are important: testosterone and its active metabolites oestradiol and dihydrotestosterone exert a profound suppressive effect upon both LH and FSH section.
- The Sertoli cell also produces other substances, termed activins, which have a stimulatory effect upon pituitary FSH secretion.
- Oestrogens probably have similar functions to androgens, but it is not known why the stallion reproduces such large quantities of these hormones, i.e. 17 β-oestradiol sulphate and oestrone sulphate.
- Circulating blood concentrations of testosterone and oestrogens vary considerably from hour to hour, so that measurement of a single sample is often meaningless; concentrations (particularly oestrogens) are usually highest during the breeding season.
- Stallions will usually copulate all year round, but most reproductive parameters are maximal during the breeding season.

- Non-active stallions may have lower mean testosterone concentrations than those that are mating.
- Exposure of a stallion to a mare in oestrus causes a rise in circulating oestrone sulphate concentrations within 10 minutes.
- The reproductive season can be 'brought forward', as in the mare, by increasing artificial light; in some stallions this also produces a 'premature autumn'.
- Puberty, as judged by the time when the stallion's ejaculate contains a minimum of 100×10^6 spermatozoa with at least 10% progressive motility, occurs at about 18 months; this may be influenced by the time of birth, nutritional status and breed and can be considerably delayed in certain individuals.

25.3 PHYSIOLOGY OF SPERM PRODUCTION

The testis is composed of a network of small tubes (the seminiferous tubules), in which spermatozoa are formed; these tubules are supported by interstitial, or Leydig, cells which produce testosterone. The seminiferous tubules drain into the epididymis, where spermatozoa mature; transit along the epididymis takes approximately 10 days.

Spermatogenesis

Spermatogenesis is the process by which spermatozoa are formed; it involves multiplication of cells by division of their parents to produce the millions of spermatozoa voided in each ejaculate.

- Two forms of division occur:

  (1) Mitosis. In this case both daughter cells are exactly the same as the parent, and it is a method by which numbers are increased.
  (2) Meiosis. This is a complicated and important division in which genetic material is firstly 'shuffled', and then halved; this latter process is essential so that each spermatozoon carries 32 chromosomes. The ovum from the mare will also contain 32 chromosomes (half the number in normal horse cells) so that combination of the two at fertilisation will produce a new individual with 64 chromosomes in each cell.

- Spermatogenesis is therefore a very complicated process; the whole process from parent cell to spermatozoon takes about 50 days.
- Spermatozoa may be ejaculated from 14 months of age and puberty generally occurs between 14 and 24 months.
- Maximum reproductive capacity is generally not reached until 4 years of age.
- Daily spermatozoal production is usually stable from 4 years to 20 years of age.
- After 20 years reproductive senescence may occur.

Ejaculate

The ejaculate is the total material emitted from the stallion's penis during coitus; this is usually achieved by six to nine urethral contractions, each one producing a jet of semen.

- The ejaculate is composed of:

  (1) spermatozoa: there are enough spermatozoa in the ductus deferens (including ampulla) for each ejaculation. Most of the spermatozoa (80%) are contained within the first three jets of the ejaculate
  (2) seminal plasma: this is provided by the accessory glands (prostate, bulb-urethral and seminal vesicles) and is the medium in which the spermatozoa are suspended. It also acts as a temporary energy source.

- Some stallions produce large quantities of gelatinous material (gel) from the seminal vesicles; this is emitted in the latter part of the ejaculate and its function is unknown, although it can make semen evaluation difficult (**26.4**).

Normal semen

The quality of horse semen is influenced by many factors, including season of year and frequency of ejaculation. In general the higher values for the parameters measured occur in the summer, in horses that are used sparingly. However, there is no absolute link between semen quality and fertility (**27.1**).

- Stallions over four years old have greater spermatozoa reserves than younger horses.
- Stallions with large testes generally produce more spermatozoa, although there is some debate about the absolute relationship.
- The tail of the epididymis is the major site of spermatozoa storage and contains more than 60% of extragonadal spermatozoal reserves.
- The rate of ejaculation does not affect spermatozoal transit time through the epididymis.
  NB: Stallions with values lower than those quoted above are not necessarily infertile or sterile (**27.1**).

25.4 MATING BEHAVIOUR (see also Chapter 6)

Pasture breeding

- Contrary to popular belief, stallions that run constantly with mares rarely get seriously kicked.
- In the early breeding season, feral stallions tend to 'herd' their band of mares to keep them in a group.
- The stallion can recognise, however, those mares that are in heat,

possibly visually (by the attitude they adopt when they are near him) or by smell.
- The stallion will not try to mate mares that are not in oestrus.
- Mares that are in heat may get mated several times a day, particularly at dawn and dusk.
- Stallions show a preference for some mares and may ignore other mares that are well in heat.
- The restrictions on pasture breeding are that infections are hard to deal with, conception dates may be difficult to ascertain and the stallion will only be able to mate with a small number of mares (about 15).

Breeding 'in hand'

- Exposure of stallions to mares only when they are ready to be mated induces a conditioned response.
- Usually the stallion knows when he is approaching the mating area, as opposed to being taken out to be lunged, ridden, shod, etc.
- The stallion's excitement is evidenced by vocalisation, rearing, bucking and trying to get close to the mare; the extent to which he becomes difficult to handle at this time depends on the individual horse, the way he has been trained and the competence of the present handler.
- When confronted with a mare in heat the stallion should:

  (1) achieve an erection. This may occur before the stallion sees the mare, after a short period of vigorous 'teasing' of the mare or, in some horses, after an extremely long wait (**27.8**)
  (2) tease the mare by vocalising, licking, holding her tail in his teeth, nuzzling the vulva, nipping or biting
  (3) exhibit flehmen, i.e. curl his lip upwards and extend his head and neck forward and upwards. Stallions do this more frequently when in the presence of an oestrus, compared with a non-oestrus mare, but mares, geldings and foals also do it occasionally. It is thought that this posture enhances the possibility of pheromones reaching the vomeronasal organ; sometimes mare's urine is seen to run into the stallion's nose, but often it doesn't
  (4) mount the mare. He may try to do this immediately on contacting the mare, with or without erection, or after a variable period of teasing. Correct early training is necessary to ensure that the stallion mounts at the right time
  (5) gain intromission, followed by thrusting.

Intromission

- Most stallions gain intromission without help, and some resent having their penis touched; however, help may be necessary, particularly if the mare's vulva has been sutured or is of an abnormal shape (**6.7**, **13.2**) (it is essential to check that the stallion has not entered the mare's rectum – thrusting within the rectum may cause a rectal tear).

- After gaining intromission, the stallion usually starts to ejaculate in 15–30 seconds but occasionally:

  (1) this can be almost immediate and can be missed by the handler
  (2) some stallions dismount without having ejaculated; on average stallions require 1.5–2 mounts to achieve ejaculation.

Ejaculation

Ejaculation is recognised by:

- cessation of thrusting
- 'flagging', i.e. the stallion's tail pumps up and down; this may be difficult to recognise if the stallion is mating a tall mare as he may also be moving his tail from side to side as he shifts weight from one foot to another
- feeling urethral pulses on the ventral surface of the penis
- observing the stallion when he has dismounted; a stallion that has ejaculated usually loses his erection and is not interested in the mare for a least a few minutes. A stallion that hasn't ejaculated usually remains keen and regains his erection rapidly (if it is lost) and re-mounts the mare. However, stallions with poor libido may lose interest without having ejaculated (**27.8**).

Dismount

- As described above; this may not indicate that the stallion has ejaculated.
- If ejaculation has occurred, the stallion may dismount:

  (1) during ejaculation – in most cases the material which is lost is the viscous seminal vesicle secretion
  (2) after ejaculation but before loss of erection
  (3) after both ejaculation and loss of erection.

26 Examination of the Stallion for Breeding Soundness

26.1 BACTERIOLOGICAL SWABBING (see also 14.1)

Rationale

- In most sexually transmitted bacterial diseases of horses, the stallion is purely a carrier, i.e. he shows no signs of infection and is not affected in any way.
- The organisms usually thrive as commensals in the sites where smegma accumulates.
- Occasionally bacteria can be isolated from the internal genitalia (e.g. pathogenic *Klebsiella*).
- Routine screening of stallions (for carriers of these venereal organisms) is therefore desirable.

Requirements

- Different breed societies have different requirements, and these are usually related to the value of the horses involved.
- The Code of Practice for the control of venereal disease (Appendix) in the United Kingdom, Ireland, France and Germany requires that all Thoroughbred stallions have two sets of swabs taken yearly, between 1 January and the start of the breeding season.
- It is only logical for any stud which requires mares to have had clitoral swabs taken before mating also to have had their stallions swabbed.
- A minimum requirement on any stud should be one set of swabs.
- The interval of one year between swabbing is arbitrary but fits in with the horse's normal breeding cycle; however, in cases of otherwise inexplicable infertility or known cases of venereal disease, extra swabs should be taken where appropriate.
- The Code of Practice recommends swabbing stallions from the urethra, urethral fossa (including the urethral diverticulum) and the sheath; it also suggests collection of pre-ejaculatory fluid.
- It is also logical (but not required) to swab at the end of the breeding season.

Technique

- In order to swab a stallion properly, his penis must be 'drawn' (exposed).
- This may be achieved by:

  (1) administering tranquillisers, e.g. acetylpromazine, xylazine or detomidine.
  NB: the possibility of the stallion being unable to retract his penis after these drugs, especially the phenothiazines, should be borne in mind and discussed with the owner beforehand. If unavoidable, xylazine is probably the drug of choice. Such a method generally precludes the possibility of collecting pre-ejaculatory fluid, although some stallions exhibit passive ejaculation when given α_2-adrenoceptor agonists (like xylazine or detomidine)
  (2) teasing the stallion with a mare so that he achieves an erection; this may include allowing the stallion to mount an oestrus mare.

The method that the author favours (finds least dangerous) is the following:

- Have a mare, not necessarily in heat, restrained at the back of a loose box.
- Allow the stallion, in the yard, to tease the mare over the box door.
- Invariably the stallion puts his head into the doorway which reduces the likelihood of his rearing, bucking, moving sideways or observing the Veterinary Surgeon.
- Once the horse is drawn, even if he hasn't achieved a full erection, running the hand over the horse's side and belly and holding the penis is usually not resented.
- The Veterinary Surgeon standing on the horse's left, holds the penis in his left (gloved) hand; either three swabs can be held in the right hand, each protruding through a different finger space, or successive swabs can be passed by an assistant.
- Passage of a swab into the urethra, and manipulation of a swab in the fossa and diverticulum are rarely noticed by the stallion.
- Pushing the third swab into the preputial fold, at the base of the penis, should be carried out last as this often provokes the stallion to kick.
- These swabs are more likely to pick up dry material, particularly that from the prepuce, if previously moistened; this can be done by dipping into sterile water (*not* saline) or into the Amie's transport medium, before use.
- Swabs are immediately placed in the transport medium before being sent to the laboratory.

26.2 PHYSICAL EXAMINATION

Observation

Observation of the stallion mating a mare is not always practical, but where possible should include the following:

- Reaction of stallion to mare – is he genuinely interested (i.e. not just noisy and physical)?
- Does he gain an erection within a reasonable time?
- Does he mount properly and thrust?
- Can he gain intromission (given that the mare is normal)?
- Does he ejaculate (as judged by palpation of the urethra)?
- Does he withdraw before ejaculation is complete?

Examination of external genitalia

Penis

This is observed prior to mating; irregularities may be due to haematomata, tumours or other lesions (see later).

Scrotum and contents

These are more easily examined after the stallion has ejaculated; abnormalities that may be detected may include:

- lesions in the scrotal skin
- disparity in size of testes or epididymides (**27.3**)
- abnormal position of a testis; rotation through 90 to 180° probably doesn't affect spermatogenesis and may be corrected manually.

Examination of the internal genitalia **per rectum**

This is usually only carried out in cases of infertility, although routine examination, including ultrasonography, may be rewarding.

26.3 SEMEN COLLECTION (also see 24.1)

The artificial vagina (AV)

- Several models are available, but all rely on the basic principles shown in Fig. 26.1.
- Most AVs have a closed collecting system, although some are open ended and semen jets have to be 'caught'.
- Basically there is an outer rigid tube and an inner soft liner (this may be plastic or latex); the space between these is filled with warm water.
- The collecting system is arranged so that semen contacts the latex liner for the shortest time possible, i.e. enters the collecting vessel immediately.

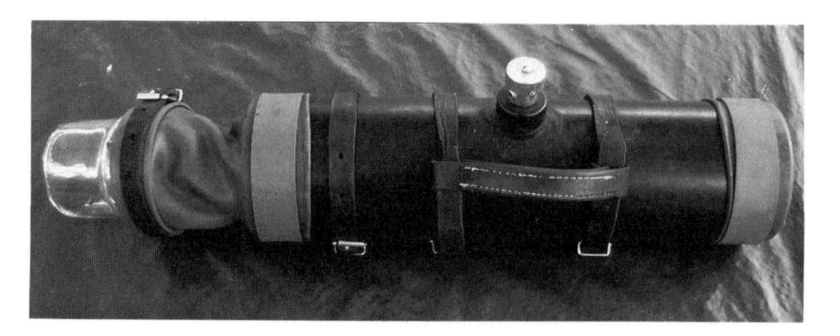

Fig. 26.1. One type of artificial vagina for collecting stallion semen.

- In cold conditions a system of lagging the collecting vessel is desirable to prevent temperature shock to the spermatozoa.
- Most AVs incorporate a filter (surgical gauze or double thickness tissue) which holds back the gelatinous seminal vesicle secretion, but allows passage of the spermatozoa rich fraction (**25.3**).
  NB: A significant number of spermatozoa are lost in the liner and in the filter.
- Water at 50–52°C is introduced into the AV, to provide a temperature in the lumen of about 44°C.
- The AV liner is lubricated with a small volume of non-spermicidal substance (most lubricants are toxic to spermatozoa, the most toxic being water soluble lubricants, and the least toxic being fat soluble lubricants. The latter are, however, difficult to remove from the equipment).
- After use the liner must be cleaned meticulously, i.e. wash, rinse several times in hot running water and immerse in 70% alcohol for 20 mins; rinse with saline before use.
- The temperature in the AV will fall if there is a delay in collection; ensure that more hot water is readily available should this situation arise.
- Assessment of the amount of water which the AV should contain is difficult if the size of the stallion's penis is not known; in general it is better to overfill the AV as water can be removed quickly and this avoids the delay of having to add more.
  NB: Grossly overfilling the AV may cause it to disrupt.
- It is essential to ensure that the hole in the collecting vessel is dorsal (to avoid spillage) and left open; otherwise air forced forward by the stallion's penis cannot escape.

Collecting a sample

- Ensure that the mare holder and stallion holder know what is expected of them; consider wearing protective clothing.
- Select a quiet mare that is well in heat and restrain her adequately. The mare's tail should be bandaged.

- Stand on the same side as the stallion handler (left) and allow the stallion to mount.
- Immediately deflect the erect penis to the side of the mare and introduce it into the AV; this may be difficult due to thrusting of the stallion and movement of the mare.
- Always be prepared for the mare to kick or turn, or for the stallion to dismount.
- Once the penis is in the AV, keep the collecting vessel lower than the other end so that ejaculate flows freely into the vessel.
- If the stallion is reluctant to thrust, it may be necessary for the collector to manipulate the AV over the stallion's penis.
- Ejaculation is recognised by appearance of fluid in the collecting vessel (if not lagged), urethral contractions or flagging.
- If the stallion dismounts during late ejaculation, be prepared to let more water out of the AV to prevent the fully erect penis from sticking inside the AV.

  NB: Temperatures in the lumen of the AV in excess of 50°C could damage spermatozoa.

26.4 SEMEN EVALUATION

The equipment necessary for semen evaluation should have been assembled before collection, but does not need to be elaborate; basically it is essential to have a microscope, microscope slides, cover slips, pipettes, a method of keeping the sample warm (water bath), a method of keeping the microscope slides warm and vital stain, e.g. nigrosin/eosin – also of use are semen extender and buffered formal saline. The various assessments, and means by which they are evaluated, are as follows:

Volume

This can be measured using the collection vessel. If this is not possible the ejaculate must be transferred to a suitable (warmed) measuring device.

- Ejaculate volume is normally 60–70 ml, but this may vary between 30 and 300 ml depending upon the size of the stallion and the season of the year.
- The volume of gel fraction may also vary.

Colour

- The normal ejaculate is pale white, similar to skimmed milk in appearance.
- There is not normally contamination with blood or urine which will cause discoloration. If the sample is discoloured examination of stained semen smears (e.g. using the modified Wright–Giemsa stain, Diff-Quik) may allow identification of contaminating cellular material such as red blood cells, or white blood cells.

Spermatozoal concentration

This can be measured using:

- An electronic counting chamber which has been calibrated to count cells of this size. This is often inaccurate since spermatozoa tails may lodge across the orifice of the device.
- A colorimeter previously calibrated for stallion semen. This has obvious inaccuracies.
- A haemocytometer counting chamber, after suitable dilution of the sample:

  (1) a proportion of the semen is well mixed and is diluted 1 in 200 with distilled water containing a little detergent (to prevent spermatozoal clumping)
  (2) one drop is placed into the chamber which has a standard depth and a known grid engraved upon its surface. Counting the number of spermatozoa within the grid (known area therefore known volume), allows calculation of the original spermatozoal concentration. It is customary to count squares diagonally across the grid. Normal values are between 100×10^6 and 800×10^6/ml.

Total spermatozoal output

This is a more meaningful measure than concentration or volume alone. Normal stallions produce between 4×10^9 and 14×10^9 spermatozoa within each ejaculate.

Percentage motility

The vessel containing the semen must be placed immediately into a water bath at approximately 37°C to prevent cooling. A drop of semen is then placed onto a warmed microscope slide and covered with a cover slip. The slide is best kept warm by housing the slide in a thermostatically controlled stage, or keeping the slide on a flat-sided medicine bottle which has been filled with warm water; evaluation at low temperatures will give erroneous results.

- The sample should be assessed under low and high power magnification.
- The assessment of motility is subjective, but the same observer can become very consistent.
- Samples should be assessed for the percentage of progressive motility. It is often easiest to categorise spermatozoal motility, using five groups:

  Category 0 – non motile spermatozoa
  Category I – spermatozoa that are motile but not progressive
  Category II – spermatozoa that are motile but poorly progressive
  Category III – spermatozoa that are motile but moderately progressive
  Category IV – spermatozoa that are motile and rapidly progressive (swimming quickly in a forward direction).

Using these criteria normal stallions have more than 50% spermatozoa with Category IV motility.

Morphology

This is the percentage of spermatozoa that conform to the shape accepted as normal for stallion semen.

- Morphology can be examined in wet preparations, but in general fixation and staining of the sperm is necessary.
- A variety of stains have been described including Giemsa.
- A simple method may be used that allows spermatozoal morphology and membrane integrity to be established at the same time; this is called vital staining.
- Vital staining uses a simple stain, nigrosin– eosin that is best refrigerated between use:

  (1) The eosin is taken up by cells that were dead at the time of staining (damaged membranes), and they therefore appear pink.
  (2) The nigrosin provides a background stain so that the spermatozoa are silhouetted against it and their shape can be seen. Nigrosin has a purple–blue colour.
  (3) Spermatozoa that appear white are classified as live. These sperm have intact membranes which prevent the eosin from penetrating into the sperm.
  NB: The head of the spermatozoa is bilaterally flattened like a table tennis bat.

- A suggested method of preparing a vital smear is as follows:

  (1) Pipette six drops of stain into a test tube in the water bath and leave for 1–2 minutes for the temperature to equilibrate.
  (2) Add one drop of semen; this ratio will allow a sample of average concentration to provide a field with spermatozoa close enough to observe conveniently, without them lying on top of each other.
  (3) Shake gently to mix, and immediately transfer one drop with a clean pipette to one of two waiting slides; smear the drop as for a blood film with a third slide and with the material left adherent to the latter make another smear on the second slide.
  (4) By experience it will become clear which smear is easier to view under the microscope, but usually it is the second.
  (5) Allow the smear to dry (about 1 minute) and assess its quality under high power ($\times$ 40 objective lens); if cells are reasonably spaced for evaluation change to oil immersion lens and record 100 cells.
  NB: It is normal for the mid-piece to be attached to the side of the neck (abaxial mid piece) and stallion spermatozoa have asymmetrical heads of varying shapes.
  (6) The main classifications of spermatozoa will be (Fig. 26.2):

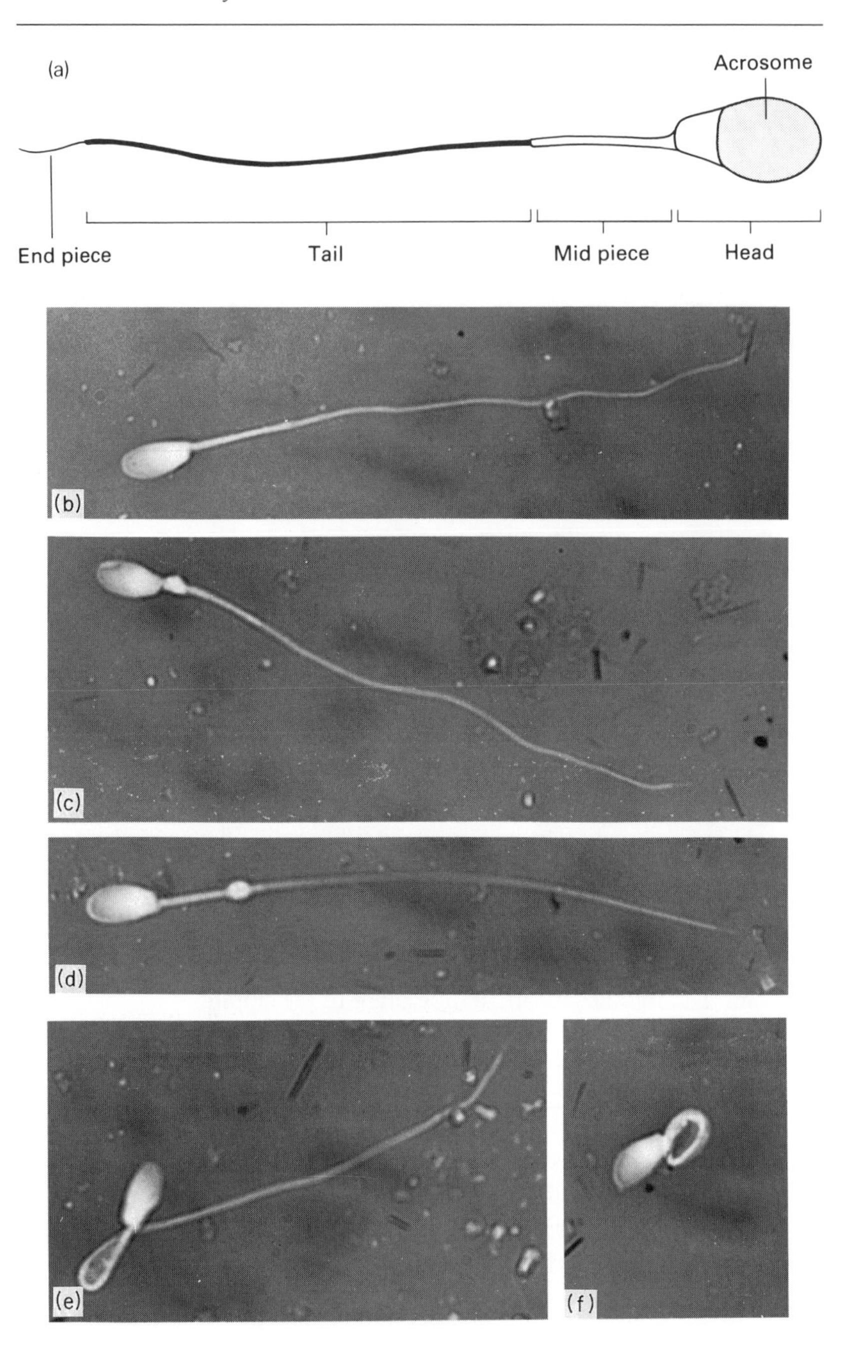

Fig. 26.2. (a) Diagram of a normal stallion spermatozoon. Stallion spermatozoa: (b) normal; (c) proximal cytoplasmic droplet and acrosomal defect; (d) distal cytoplasmic droplet and separating acrosome; (e) bent mid-piece; (f) coiled mid-piece and tail and separating acrosome; (g) knobbed acrosome.

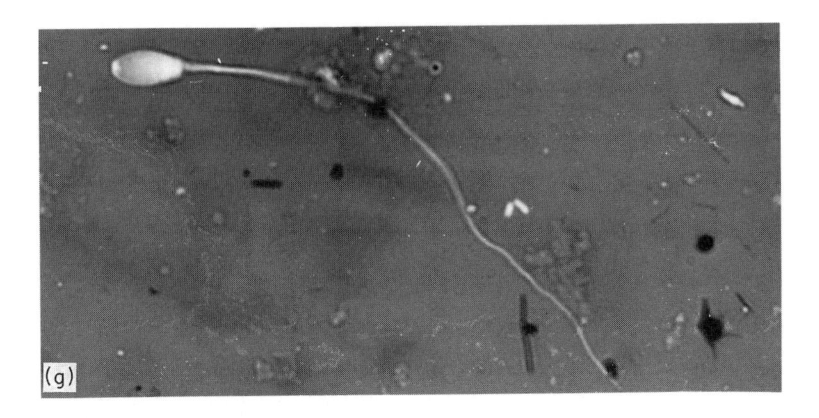

normal – live
normal – dead
separated head (dead)
knobbed acrosome
oedematous acrosome
detached acrosome
crater defect
neck tags or mid piece disruption } live
proximal cytoplasmic droplet } live
distal cytoplasmic droplet
bent mid piece
coiled tail
looped tail

(7) Normal live spermatozoa and those with a distal cytoplasmic droplet (which is a remnant of the cytoplasm left after the spermatozoa's metamorphosis from a spermatid, and is used as an indication of spermatozoal maturity) are added and represent the percentage of spermatozoa which are considered normal. More detailed examination of 'normal' spermatozoa are using different stains or electron microscopy may reveal previously unrecognised abnormalities.

- Other tests. A variety of other tests are now used to assess spermatozoa, including the hypo-osmotic swelling test (a test of functional integrity of the spermatozoal membrane), and spermatozoal penetration assays.
- ALWAYS put some of the sample into buffered formal saline (roughly 1:1), wax the bottle cap to prevent evaporation and label the bottle clearly; this provides for retrospective checking in any cases of doubt. NB: It has become customary to evaluate two samples collected one hour apart.

26.5 WHEN SHOULD SEMEN BE EVALUATED?

- Routinely each year before the breeding season (may also be done to estimate optimum number of mares that can be mated per season).
- When lowered fertility is suspected.
- When abnormal sexual behaviour is seen.
- If a pathogenic infection is suspected.
- Before sale.
- For semen preservation and artificial insemination.

27 Infertility in the Stallion

27.1 POOR SEMEN QUALITY

Defining the problem

- The words 'fertile', 'infertile' and 'subfertile' are all relative and describe different degrees of being able to get mares in foal.
- The term 'sterile' denotes complete inability to breed, as in a castrate.
- The quality of semen below which a stallion has reduced fertility cannot be defined and will, amongst other things, depend on the number of times that he is used.
- It is surprising that stallions with very poor motility and/or morphology of spermatozoa will still get a small percentage of mares in foal.
- The results of semen evaluation can only be interpreted in conjunction with other information; the only proof of fertility is that the stallion mated a mare (which was not mated by another stallion at the same heat), and that she was either unequivocally found to be in foal by a method that reliably aged the pregnancy, or produced a foal at the expected time after mating.
- However, as a guideline, it has been suggested that stallions with seminal values consistently above the following should not have fertility problems; gel-free volume of ejaculate 25 ml; spermatozoal concentration 20×10^6/ml; total spermatozoa output 1.3×10^9; total live spermatozoa output 1.1×10^9.

Causes

- The causes of poor seminal quality, in the absence of other obvious disease processes, are poorly understood. Some possible contributing factors are:

  (1) Pyrexia. Any disease which causes a rise in temperature is likely to cause a disruption in spermatogenesis; however, due to antibiotics, it is unusual for such a condition to exist for any length of time. Normal spermatozoa should appear in the ejaculate 2 months after recovery.

(2) Anabolic steroids. These drugs are most likely to be given to horses in training; they depress spermatogenesis but after withdrawal of these drugs this process returns to normal after about 3 months.
(3) Over use. Most stallions can mate 15 times a week without a reduction of seminal quality; however, some stallions may not be able to cope with this regime. In normal stallions the third ejaculation of the day is as fertile as the first.
(4) Very rarely a stallion may produce an ejaculate of poor quality, followed 1–2 hours later by a 'normal' ejaculate; it is thus desirable to collect twice from a stallion during a fertility examination.
(5) Nutritional factors may affect semen quality but these have not been described fully.
(6) Masturbation. There is no evidence that this reduces fertility.
(7) Some stallions produce a higher number of abnormal spermatozoa after a long sexual rest.

NB: It is usually suggested that semen evaluation is carried out after the stallion has rested for 5–7 days; however, for a busy stallion this may give a false impression of seminal quality.
NB: The quality of the ejaculate reflects the conditions of spermatogenesis 60 days previously.

Treatment

Management
If a management factor is identified it must be corrected and if the problem appears to be recent it is worth testing again in two months time.

Teasing
This may decrease the reaction time and increase the volume of accessory secretion but has no effect on spermatozoal output.

Hormones
There is no evidence that hormone treatment, e.g. gonadotrophins or gonadotrophin releasing hormone, has any affect on semen quality. The use of steroid hormones is contraindicated since these have a negative feedback effect upon the hypothalamus/pituitary axis (**25.2**).

27.2 INFECTIONS (see also Chapters 13–16)

General considerations

- Active infection of the stallion's genital tract, giving rise to recognisable lesions, are rare (e.g. orchitis, epididymitis, seminal vesiculitis).
- Two viral conditions occur, i.e. coital exanthema, which is self-limiting, and equine viral arteritis (**16.3**).

- Stallions can be carriers of venereal organisms; they show no signs of disease, but spread the organisms from mare to mare. It is only this latter situation which will be considered further.

Diagnosis

- This usually occurs when pre-breeding season swabs are taken from the stallion's penis or sheath; swabs may also be taken at other times if an infectious fertility problem is suspected (**26.1**).
- The organisms which are considered dangerous are *Taylorella equigenitalis*, *Klebsiella pneumoniae* (capsule types 1, 2 and 5) and *Pseudomonas aeruginosa*.
- Only some strains of *P. aeruginosa* appear to be pathogenic but these cannot be identified chemically or serologically; it may be necessary to test-mate two or three mares and observe them closely for signs of endometritis.
- Some stallions have been known to excrete *K. pneumoniae* or *P. aeruginosa* in the ejaculate and not harbour the organism on the penis; the site of bacterial multiplication has not been found.
- Mycoplasmata and fungi are found in the ejaculate of many stallions but their significance is unknown.

Treatment

- Do not wash the stallion's penis routinely with antiseptics as these increase the incidence of resistant pseudomonads.
- For stallions which ejaculate bacteria, parenteral gentamycin (4.4 mg/kg twice daily) or neomycin (3 g twice daily) are effective.
- In general, however, systemic treatment is not necessary and the following local regime should be adopted:

  (1) The stallion's penis must be exposed by teasing him with a mare, or administering sedatives (**26.1**).
  (2) The penis and sheath must be washed thoroughly with warm water and soft soap; attention must be paid to removing smegma from the sheath and the urethral fossa and sinus.
  (3) Do not use chlorhexidine; there is evidence that this can be absorbed locally and can interfere with spermatogenesis. However, diluted hydrochloric or acetic acid may be useful for reducing pseudomonads, and diluted sodium hypochlorite may be useful for certain *Klebsiella* spp.
  (4) Dry the penis well.
  (5) Apply any of the following:
      an antibiotic ointment based upon sensitivity; those containing neomycin, polymyxin and furazolidine are often the most effective
      silver sulphadiazine cream; this has been used to clear pseudo-

monad organisms in particular
silver nitrate as a 1% spray

(6) Repeat the washing, drying and antiseptic routine daily for five days.
(7) If swabs are negative for venereal organisms, a bacteriological broth containing the normal flora of the stallion's penis (e.g. non-haemolytic streptococci, *Streptococcus faecalis*, diphtheroids, staphylococci, etc.) is applied daily for five days.

- If subsequent swabs are positive, cleansing treatment should be continued.
- If bacteria cannot be eliminated from a stallion's ejaculate mares can be inseminated or the minimal contamination technique can be used (**15.2**).

27.3 DISEASES OF THE TESTES AND SCROTUM

Neoplasia

Testicular tumours are rare; seminomas and teratomas appear to be the commonest. A higher incidence of neoplasia is noted in abdominal testes (cryptorchidism). Usually the affected testis enlarges but is not painful. Diagnosis may be made by biopsy, although this may severely disrupt the normal testicular function. A more suitable method is ultrasound examination. Metastases are rare.

Abnormal position of the testes (cryptorchidism) (see also 28.3)

This may be either unilateral or bilateral. Unilateral cryptorchids are more common. May be defined as inguinal (temporary or permanent), or abdominal (complete or incomplete). Generally these are presented to the Veterinary Surgeon as:

(1) owned since a foal and no history of surgery – diagnosis is easy
(2) presented for castration with one scrotal testis – further investigation is required
(3) presented as a gelding but behaving as if entire – further investigation is required.

Unilateral cryptorchids are fertile but should not be used for breeding. The congenital presence of a single testis within the body (monorchidism) is extremely rare, and congenital absence (anorchidism) even rarer.

Hypoplasia

This is rare, may be congenital or acquired and cases are usually presented as bilaterally small testes. The testicular parenchyma has reduced echogenicity when examined with ultrasound. There is no treatment.

Testicular degeneration

This condition is usually an acquired condition secondary to thermal injury (generalised or localised), toxins, or autoantibodies. Semen quality is poor and the testes are usually of abnormal size and texture. Testicular biopsy may be useful for its diagnosis but this causes testicular damage, and is not useful for assessment of prognosis. In early cases damage may be minimised by reducing the testicular temperature. The prognosis is guarded once changes are established.

Torsion of the spermatic cord

This causes rotation of the testis around its dorsal axis. In some cases the epididymis may be palpated in the lateral or cranial part of the scrotum; torsion through 180 degrees may neither cause signs of discomfort nor infertility, and may be reduced manually. In severe cases of torsion, abdominal pain and marked swelling result; prompt removal of the swollen testis may be necessary to prevent testicular degeneration of the remaining testicle (because of the local swelling and oedema).

Orchitis

The most common cause of testicular inflammation is local trauma (kicks, etc.). In a few cases this may result in subsequent immune mediated orchitis when there is breakdown of the blood–testis barrier. Infective orchitis may result from a penetrating wound or from haematogenous spread (streptococci for example). Viral orchitis may be caused by EVA. In all cases there is usually swelling and pain, and treatment is aimed at controlling the primary cause and attempting to reduce the testicular temperature to prevent subsequent testicular degeneration.

Testicular haematoma

These usually result from traumatic lesions, and control of swelling and heat is the primary aim to prevent subsequent testicular degeneration.

Scrotal hernia

This is uncommon but may be confused with orchitis. Ultrasound examination of the scrotum, or rectal palpation of the inguinal region may confirm the presence of abdominal contents within the scrotum.

Adhesions

Adhesions between the parietal and visceral layers of the tunica vaginalis restrict the movement of the testis in the scrotum. These are signs of previous scrotal/testicular disease.

27.4 DISEASES OF THE PENIS AND SHEATH

Coital exanthema

Caused by EHV3 (**16.2**), and results in the presence of small vesicles on the penis and sheath. These usually resolve spontaneously within a few weeks, but the stallion may be unwilling to mate during this time because of the inflammation.

Bacterial infections

The common pathogenic venereal bacteria do not cause clinical disease in the stallion.

Phimosis (small preputial orifice)

This may be either a congenital stricture of the prepuce, or the result of an enlarged penis (inflammation, neoplastic invasion). In either case it may cause urine pooling and dribbling, and surgical treatment may be required.

Paraphimosis (failure to retract the penis)

This may be the result of:

- trauma during breeding (haematoma)
- a complication of castration (not an effect of the sedative agent)
- phenothiazine tranquillisers
- neuromuscular disease.

In cases of traumatic paraphimosis, the free part of the penis is swollen; the preputial part is most swollen and thus points backwards. Initial treatment is to establish whether the horse can urinate by placing him into a clean box, or by rectal examination to detect a full bladder. If the condition is seen early, aim to reduce the size of the penis by using a pressure bandage and massage. Otherwise prevent gravity oedema by supporting the penis (a towel placed under the penis and tied over the stallion's back). Clean the penis daily and apply lubricant. Eventually the oedema subsides and the penis can be replaced. If the penile skin splits, the oedema fluid is lost and the penis can be replaced. Support may be necessary for up to three weeks in certain cases. Surgery is unlikely to be necessary. Never operate on an oedematous penis, it will not heal.

Priapism (persistent enlargement without sexual excitement)

Generally the result of phenothiazine tranquillisers. If the penis is turgid and not retracted, push it back and place towel clips or sutures across the prepuce. Remove these after 12 hours and recheck the penis. If the priapism is permanent, amputation may be necessary. It is advisable to avoid the use of these agents in stallions.

Penile neoplasia

Not uncommon, frequently seen in older geldings – smegma is carcinogenic. Squamous cell carcinoma is the most common tumour. It frequently arises within the urethral diverticulae, and there may be kissing lesions onto the preputial ring. These are often small pink cauliflower-like lesions. White depigmented plaques may represent pre-tumorous changes. Tumours are generally noticed when there is haemorrhage from the lesion or when the lesion is very large. Treatment is via penile amputation and removal of the preputial ring ('reefing'). The prognosis is good if treated early, but tumours may metastasise to the inguinal lymph nodes.

27.5 DISEASES OF THE INTERNAL GENITALIA

- Diseases of the prostate gland are extremely rare.
- Seminal vesiculitis is rare. Common causes are bacterial invasion. Several bacteria may be isolated including *Klebsiella* and *Pseudomonas*. There are often few clinical signs; usually only changes in semen quality, including reduced spermatozoal longevity and the presence of blood and/or pus. Stallions may become persistently infected resulting in reduced fertility, or they may infect mares (especially if the primary bacterium is *Klebsiella* or *Pseudomonas*). Treatment is difficult as there is poor penetration of antibiotics. Endoscopic lavage and antibiotic packing, or surgical ablation, may be attempted but these are technically difficult.

27.6 ABNORMALITIES OF THE EJACULATE

Haemospermia

This has been associated with a significant reduction in fertility. It appears that the effect is due to whole blood not serum; the mechanism is unknown. The condition may be the result of:

- bacterial urethritis
- laceration of the penis
- accessory gland infection

Traumatic lesions generally heal with sexual rest. However, treatment of urethritis and accessory gland infections may necessitate the use of urinary acidifiers and systemic antibiotics. In certain cases a temporary subischial urethrostomy with package of the urethra with antibiotic and steroid may be needed for the treatment of urethritis.

Urospermia

This may result in infertility but not always. Some cases are the result of sphincter mechanism incompetence or other neuropathies (e.g. EHV1).

Management may include mating or semen collection after urination, semen collection and immediate dilution in a semen extender, or the possible use of α_1-adrenoceptor agonists.

27.7 ABNORMALITIES OF MATING

- Failure to achieve an erection could be due to the presence of a stallion ring (fitted to prevent masturbation); but see also psychological infertility.
- Failure to ejaculate. This may also be psychological, but in some cases the stallion is thought to have ejaculated purely because he has dismounted. Ejaculation can be confirmed by observing flagging, feeling urethral pulses and observing the stallion after dismounting; in most cases a stallion which has ejaculated will retract his penis and show little interest in the mare, but some will mount and ejaculate again.
- Retrograde ejaculation. Ejaculation into the urinary bladder; if signs of ejaculation occur but the ejaculate is incomplete, it is possible that some has passed forwards and into the bladder. Examination of a voided urine sample will aid the diagnosis.
- Blind stallions may have problems mounting.
- Mounting and/or thrusting may be prevented by painful conditions, e.g. trauma, cauda equina neuritis, ilio-femoral thrombosis, laminitis, arthritis, coital exanthema; the administration of analgesics may alleviate the condition.
- Overuse. The stallion may have reduced libido; however, this is an unlikely cause of infertility in normal stallions as:

  (1) there is evidence that the first, second and third ejaculations of the day are equally fertile
  (2) although collecting semen hourly for five ejaculations causes a decrease in volume and total spermatozoa output, the percentage of normal and motile spermatozoa remains the same.

27.8 PSYCHOLOGICAL PROBLEMS

- These account for a large proportion of infertility in stallions and usually arise because of the way the stallion has been managed.
- There is often a thin line between the discipline required to manage a strong young healthy stallion, and that which acts as aversion therapy.
- Some stallions may have been kicked by mares, particularly when young.

Signs of psychological infertility

- Complete disinterest in mares, or very long reaction time; this may occur with all mares, or only some individuals, mares of a particular colour or those with foals at foot.

- Inability to gain an erection (suspect a stallion ring).
- Inability to mount (may be physical).
- Inability to thrust (may be physical).
  NB: If the mare has air in her vagina, e.g. after a speculum examination, a normal stallion will not be stimulated to thrust.
- Inability to ejaculate after repeated thrusting and mounting.
- Dismounting at the beginning of ejaculation (may be physical, e.g. due to urethritis).
- Inability to mate with more than one mare every day or every two days.
- A stallion frustrated in one of the above ways may often become very vicious towards the mare and may try to kick at the mare or handler.
- Some impotent stallions have normal testosterone, but lowered oestradiol, luteinising hormone and follicle stimulating hormone concentrations – it is not known if this is cause or effect.
- Anabolic steroids do not reduce sexual drive.

Treatment of psychological infertility

- The therapist must be prepared to spend a lot of time with these stallions, and to be patient.
- A specific diagnosis may never be arrived at, but the following suggestions may help to correct the problem:

  (1) Observe the stallion's behaviour with its usual handler, and then with a complete (experienced) stranger.
  (2) Run the stallion with an experienced mare that is well in oestrus.
  (3) Allow the stallion to watch another horse mate with a mare with which he has failed.
  (4) Restrain another horse (i.e. potential competitor) close to the problem stallion and mare; if successful this 'observer' may become a specific requirement.
  (5) Cover the mare's rump (particularly if the stallion shows a mare preference) with the stallion's faeces or the urine of another mare that is in oestrus.
  (6) Limit the number of matings of stallions which cannot ejaculate regularly.
  (7) Diazepam, 0.05 mg/kg intravenously, 5–10 minutes before mating has been found to be beneficial in some stallions.
  (8) Placing the non-erect penis in a warm artificial vagina, even if the stallion has not mounted, may stimulate sexual arousal – this can be progressively converted into normal coital behaviour.
  (9) Although in the normal stallion gonadotrophin releasing hormone administration causes an increase in luteinising hormone, follicle stimulating hormone, testosterone and oestradiol concentrations, there is no evidence that such treatment is beneficial for impotent horses.
  (10) Similarly, although administration of testosterone and oestradiol to

geldings will restore libido, impotent stallions do not benefit from this treatment and it will adversely affect spermatogenesis.

(11) Ejaculation failure may respond to noradrenaline, e.g. 0.01 mg/kg 10–15 minutes before mating.

27.9 STALLION 'VICES'

- So called vices in stallions, as in other horses, are usually caused by the boredom that results from being confined to a loose box for most of the day.
- These include box walking, weaving, crib-biting, wind-sucking, kicking, etc.
- Where stud management allows, stallions should be ridden, lunged or even turned out into a small paddock daily.
- Well exercised stallions are much easier to handle when mating.
- The use of stallion rings to stop masturbation or prevent erections during showing, etc. is to be avoided if possible.

NB: Some stallions are very dangerous; so are some mares and some geldings.

28 Miscellaneous

28.1 BREEDING TERMS

- Mare owner and stallion owner can come to any agreement they like concerning the price charged for mating the mare, and the conditions which apply to payment of the fees.
- It is always wise for both stallion owner and mare owner to be clear about the terms, and to sign documents which outline the agreement.
- Where applicable, the stage at which a mare is certified in foal, e.g. 40 days, should be stated; irrespective of historical consideration the aforementioned is a convenient time to define pregnancy for physiological reasons (**7.5**).
- As part of the agreement, the stallion owner may promise to restrict the number of mares mated by the stallion during the relevant season.
- The stallion owner may also reserve the right to refuse nominations to certain mares, e.g. maiden and old barren mares.
- Some examples of agreements are set out below:

  (1) Straight fee. This becomes payable at the end of the breeding season (15th July for Thoroughbreds) provided that the mare has been mated.
  (2) Split fee. Part of the payment is due at the end of the breeding season (whether or not the mare is certified in foal); the remainder becomes payable either on 1st October if the mare owner cannot produce a certificate from a Veterinary Surgeon to say that the mare is not in foal, or at a specified date if the mare does not produce a foal which lives for 7 days.
  (3) In some cases split fees which are due on 1st October offer an extra incentive for those who pay promptly in respect of the mare producing a viable foal (length of survival post-partum is defined).
  (4) No foal – no fee. A mare not in foal on 1st October evokes no stud fee. In some cases the stud returns the fee if no live foal is born.
  (5) No foal – free return. This provides that should a mare fail to produce a foal which lives to a specified age, the mare will be mated again by the same stallion in the next year, but thereafter renewal of the 'free return' is unlikely.

28.2 HIDDEN COSTS AT STUD

- When sending a mare to stud, the mating or stud fee is not the only expense that will be incurred.
- Incidental costs may be negligible compared with the stud fee, but the following should be anticipated:

Keep fees

These are increased if the mare has a foal at foot and should be balanced carefully with the possible benefits of travelling the mare to and from the stud and of obtaining veterinary advice.

Transportation costs

These must be incurred for travelling the mare to and from the stud once. However, if the mare is collected and taken home after mating and returned for pregnancy tests, etc., these trips should be costed.

Management costs (i.e. routine worming and foot care)

All studs must adopt a sensible worming programme and a visiting mare cannot be an exception; it is contamination of pasture which is the greatest danger to the mare (and particularly her foal).

Routine veterinary costs

Each stud adopts its own policy of vaccination against equine influenza, equine herpesvirus, equine viral arteritis and tetanus. Additionally pre-breeding genital swabbing is usually required, and newborn foals may receive antibiotics, tetanus antitoxin and regular veterinary examinations.

- These measures are part of the intense preventive medicine regime that studs must adopt in order to try to safeguard all of the animals on the premises, an individual mare and/or foal cannot be an exception.
- Attention post-foaling, i.e. examination of membranes, suturing the vulva, etc.

Specialist veterinary costs

These include:

- examination for breeding soundness
- additional uterine swabs
- examination for failure to show heat
- examination to assess readiness for mating
- prescription of hormone injections or other preparations
- treatment of uterine infections
- pregnancy diagnosis, either manual or with ultrasound (these may need to be repeated)
- management of twins.

Emergency veterinary costs

These are likely to be incurred during parturition problems or any other disease which affects either the mare or the foal.

28.3 THE 'RIGGY' GELDING

The problem

- The word 'rig' is one which is applied to cryptorchid horses, which have one or both testes undescended (still in the abdomen) (**25.1**).
- Occasionally horses that are considered to be geldings may have one (in this case the other, descended, testis has been removed by castration) or both testes in the abdomen; although these testes cannot produce spermatozoa, they do produce male hormones and the horse acts like a stallion.
- Many geldings are said to be 'riggy' because they exhibit behaviour which is interpreted as stallion-like, or because they are difficult for the owner to manage.
- The sort of behaviour that evokes the description of 'riggy' includes:

  (1) chasing or 'herding' mares or other horses in the field
  (2) obtaining an erection either in the presence of other horses or otherwise
  (3) aggression towards other horses, particularly stallions and colts
  (4) mounting mares in heat, with or without an erection
  (5) mating with mares
  (6) biting objects, people or other horses.

Possible causes of 'riggy' behaviour

- Retention of one or both abdominal testes – this can be diagnosed by hormonal tests; see next section.
- 'Cutting the horse proud', i.e. castrating the horse by removing the testis but leaving either the epididymis or a lot of the spermatic cord; this does *not* produce a true rig because:

  (1) many horses castrated in this way do not exhibit the above behaviour
  (2) growing cells from the epididymis and cord in the laboratory (tissue culture) shows that they are incapable of producing male hormones (testosterone and oestrogens)
  (3) horses which have deliberately been castrated to leave the epididymis intact do not give positive responses to the hormone tests for true cryptorchids
  (4) however, removal of the cord from previously castrated horses will sometimes improve behaviour; the mechanism by which this works is not known.

- Age of castration.

(1) In a study on the behaviour of castrated stallions, most showed a marked lack of interest in mares by 30 days after the operation.
(2) In a different study which compared the behaviour of geldings that were either castrated before two years of age, or after three years of age, it was found that in both groups 30% of the horses were less aggressive to people and 40% were less aggressive to other horses, i.e. the age of castration had no effect on aggression.
NB: This means that most geldings show some signs of aggression – and so do many mares; often the problem is managemental, including lack of confidence by the owner.

Fertility in 'rigs'

- Horses with no testes cannot be fertile.
- Cryptorchid horses are also sterile; although the testes in the abdomen can be endocrinologically active, the temperature is too high for normal spermatogenesis.
- After castration horses are usually sterile by seven days; spermatozoa may remain in the ampullae for several months but these are invariably dead and therefore not fertile.

Diagnosis of the 'true rig' (cryptorchid)

Two hormonal methods are available for the detection of testicular tissue: these are easier and cheaper than surgical exploration of the abdomen.

- Testosterone: plasma concentrations of this hormone vary so much that a single sample will not give an interpretable results. It is therefore necessary to inject the horse with a hormone which will, if normal testicular tissue is present, stimulate exaggerated testosterone production. The test procedure is: collect a heparinised blood sample for resting plasma testosterone concentration determination; inject 6000 IU human chorionic gonadotrophin (hCG) intravenously; take a second blood sample for testosterone determination 30–120 minutes after injection. A significant increase in testosterone concentration in the second sample indicates the presence of testicular tissue (functional Leydig cells).
- Oestrone sulphate: high values of this hormone indicate the presence of testicular tissue. A single blood sample taken into a heparinised container will allow assay of plasma oestrone sulphate concentrations.
  NB: This test is not suitable for horses under three years of age or for donkeys.

28.4 RECTAL TEARS

- Examination of the mare's genitalia *per rectum*, either by palpation or using ultrasound scanning, is the most commonly employed gynaecological investigation.

- This method of examination is also used in horses of all types for the investigation of other abdominal conditions, e.g. colic and cryptorchidism.
- A small, but real danger in all these examinations is that the horse's rectum may become torn, often with fatal consequences.

Some facts concerning rectal tears

- Compared with the number of horses which are examined *per rectum*, damage to the rectum wall is very infrequent.
- Rectal tears occur more often in male horses than females; this may be because:

  (1) mares become accustomed to rectal examination, but every animal must be examined for a first time
  (2) stallions and geldings may be more difficult to restrain during examination
  (3) male horses may have more 'fragile' rectums than females
  (4) the reason for rectal examination in male horses, e.g. cryptorchidism, may require more extensive abdominal exploration
  (5) in emergencies, e.g. colic, it is more likely that mares will have been previously examined by this method than male horses.

- Rectal tears happen most often during examinations by experienced practitioners.
- Rectal tears rarely occur in the area where the examiner's fingers are placed, i.e. adjacent to the structure being palpated; commonly they occur on the dorsal surface of the rectum, adjacent to the mesorectum, i.e. the lesion results from pulling the rectum away from its mesenteric attachment.
- Examiners are often unaware of rectal tears occurring, probably because they occur at the back of the hand.
- Because the usual site for rectal tears is about 30 cm cranial to the anus, and at the site of dorsal rectal attachment, it has been postulated that a 'weakness' exists in this area in some horses.
- Rectal tears can occur spontaneously.

Possible causes of rectal tears

- Application of excessive pressure to the rectal wall – this cannot be quantified but it is unlikely that an examiner will consciously evoke a rectal tear.
- Resentment of examination by the horse – during every examination the hand experiences various degrees of rectal pressure caused by involuntary peristalsis or voluntary straining; during mild peristaltic contractions examination can be continued; during strong peristaltic waves the hand should be left immobile and passive until the contraction has

passed; during forceful abdominal straining the hand should be retracted and occasionally withdrawn from the rectum.
NB: Rarely, conditions may be such that a complete examination cannot be carried out in an uncooperative animal; re-examination later, or on the next day is usually less complicated, although economical and practical considerations may make re-examination difficult.
- Sudden movements of the animal which cannot be anticipated – restraint during rectal examination is discussed in Chapter 3 and the degree adopted is usually sufficient for the examiner to feel safe. However, sudden events which may scare the mare cannot be prevented, e.g. an attendant sneezing, a car starting, a dog barking, a foal moving, etc.
- Predisposing 'weakness' of the rectal wall because of previous lesions or unknown factors.

Severity of rectal tears

Tears may be classified according to whether they are complete or incomplete, and which structures they involve. A simple classification system is in common use although it does not account for all possibilities:

(1) Grade 1 tears involve only the mucosa, or the mucosa and submucosa.
(2) Grade 2 tears involve only the muscular layers.
(3) Grade 3 tears involve the mucosa, submucosa and muscular layers.
(4) Grade 4 tears involve all layers so there is direct penetration into the peritoneal cavity.

- This classification is useful although it provides no information about the size of the defect in the rectal wall and this may also be important when considering the outcome or possible treatment options.
- The classification provides no information about the site of the rectal tear; this may be either peritoneal or retroperitoneal.
- In Grade 3 peritoneal tears the serosa or mesorectum prevents gross contamination of the peritoneal cavity; however, bacteria are not excluded and peritonitis may result.
- In Grade 4 tears there may be gross faecal contamination of the peritoneal cavity, whilst if retroperitoneal there may be cellulitis and later abscessation.
- Tears through the dorsal rectum generally enter the suspending mesentery, and this may prevent peritoneal contamination regardless of the classification of the tear.

Recognition of rectal tears

- Many rectal tears occur unknown to the examiner.
- Signs which may make the examiner suspicious that a rectal tear has occurred are:

  (1) a sudden increase in space in the rectum – this could also be due to air entering the rectum from the colon or through the anus

(2) the presence of blood on the examiner's sleeve; usually this is the result of a minor abrasion of the rectal wall or damage to the anus – in the vast majority of cases it is inconsequential. If blood is seen, a *careful* re-examination should be made; unless the examiner is aware of the usual site for rectal tears (this is unlikely to happen to any clinician more than once in his/her lifetime) a dorsal tear may be missed
(3) easily palpable viscera – when the tear is complete
(4) the development of abdominal pain and shock after rectal palpation.

- If a rectal tear is suspected, administer intravenous atropine and a low volume epidural anaesthesia. This reduces the risk of faecal contamination of the abdomen and allows careful evaluation of the position, site and severity of the tear.

Outcome of rectal tears

- Grade 1 tears generally heal without serious complication. Occasionally there may be deeper erosion and infection leading to a Grade 3 or 4 tear, although this is uncommon.
- Grade 2 tears result in a rectal diverticulum the size of which relates to the size of the initial muscular tear. The prognosis for these cases is usually good if healing is uncomplicated.
- Grade 3 and 4 tears have a poor prognosis depending upon their position and size.

Treatment of rectal tears

- Grade 1 and 2 tears are best managed conservatively. Broad spectrum antimicrobial agents should be administered, and attempts should be made to soften the faeces (lush pasture, mineral oil, etc.). Rectal palpation should be avoided for at least 1 month.
- Grade 3 and 4 tears should be initially treated by:

(1) reducing peristalsis
(2) evacuating the rectum and applying a large iodine-medicate swab to the site of the tear
(3) packing the rectum to prevent faeces entering the region of the tear.

- Primary surgical closure of tears has been described. This may be achieved either via the rectum or via a midline (or paramedian) laparotomy.
  Other techniques have been described including:

(1) diverting end or loop colostomy, which is usually performed temporarily before reconnection once the rectal tear has healed
(2) temporary indwelling rectal liner, which is usually expelled without further surgical interference.

- Surgical repair of a Grade 3 or 4 rectal tear is complicated with a high risk of failure. Due consideration should be given to the welfare and financial implications before these techniques are performed.

Reducing the likelihood of rectal tears

- Use sufficient lubricant.
- Remove all faecal material before performing the examination.
- Place your hand cranial to the structure to be palpated before moving caudally onto the structure. This tends to utilise the 'free' rectum cranially rather than the caudal rectum that is often tense.
- Do not palpate during peristaltic contractions or abdominal straining.
- If straining persists use a nose twitch.
- Consider low doses of α_2-adrenoceptor agonists in difficult animals.

Appendix: Codes of Practice on Contagious Equine Metritis (CEM), *Klebsiella pneumoniae, Pseudomonas aeruginosa*; Equine Viral Arteritis (EVA); Equid Herpesvirus-1 (EHV-1)*

INTRODUCTION

There are three Codes of Practice on:

- Contagious Equine Metritis (CEM) and infection caused by the bacteria *Klebsiella pneumoniae* and *Pseudomonas aeruginosa* †
- Equine Viral Arteritis (EVA)†
- Equid herpesvirus-1 (EHV-1)‡

† These Codes are common to Great Britain, France, Germany, Ireland and Italy.
‡ This Code is common to Great Britain and Ireland.

The Codes aim to help breeders minimise the risk of venereal disease in the horse population by making recommendations for disease prevention and control during the breeding season. Breeders should implement these minimum recommendations – and any additional precautions – in consultation with their Veterinary Surgeon.

There is a serious risk of widespread disease problems if breeders ignore the Codes. Outbreaks of reproductive disease can have severe economic and other consequences for breeding in the Thoroughbred and non-Thoroughbred sectors alike.

EVA and EHV-1 can also be transmitted by routes other than breeding and so can have severe consequences outside the breeding sector, ultimately for all branches of the horse and pony population.

* Published by the Horserace Betting Levy Board, 1996. Reprinted by kind permission of the Horserace Betting Levy Board.

Precautions are as important when using Artificial Insemination (AI) as they are for natural mating. Breeders using AI should also refer to the Code of Practice on AI published by the British Equine Veterinary Association (BEVA).

The Codes are prepared annually by a Sub-Committee of the Veterinary Advisory Committee of the Horserace Betting Levy Board. They are agreed with representatives of the other participating countries.

The Codes do not imply any liability by the Horserace Betting Levy Board or the Sub-Committee in the implementation of the recommendations nor responsibility for enforcement of the Codes.

REMEMBER:

- Breeders are responsible for implementing the Codes.
- Ignoring the Codes may jeopardise your horse(s) and those of others.
- The Codes make **minimum** recommendations for disease prevention and control.
- If using AI, refer also to the BEVA Code of Practice available from BEVA, Hartham Park, Corsham, Wiltshire SN13 0BQ.

COMMON CODE OF PRACTICE FOR CEM, *KLEBSIELLA PNEUMONIAE* AND *PSEUDOMONAS AERUGINOSA*

1. What causes these diseases?

Three species of bacteria are recognised as liable to cause outbreaks of infectious reproductive disease in the horse:

- *Taylorella equigenitalis* (CEM Organism or CEMO)
- *Klebsiella pneumoniae*
- *Pseudomonas aeruginosa*

Infection with these bacteria can be highly contagious.

2. How does infection spread?

Infection spreads through direct transmission of bacteria from mare to stallion or from stallion to mare at the time of mating. It is also transmitted to mares if semen used in AI comes from infected stallions.

Indirect infection also occurs, for example:

- through contaminated water, utensils and instruments
- on the hands of staff who handle the tail and genital area of the mare or the penis of the stallion

Indirect infection is a significant risk for the transmission of *Klebsiella pneumoniae* and *Pseudomonas aeruginosa* between horses.

3. What are the symptoms?

In the **mare**, the severity of infection with CEMO varies. The main outward clinical sign is a discharge from the vulva, resulting from inflammation of the uterus. There are three states of infection:

In the **acute** state, there is active inflammation and obvious discharge.

In the **chronic** state, the signs may be less obvious but the infection is often deep seated and may be difficult to clear.

There is also the **carrier** state. The bacteria have become established as part of the bacterial flora in the genital areas and there are no signs of infection. However, the mare is still infectious.

Infected **stallions** are usually passive carriers, meaning that they do not show clinical signs of infection but have the bacteria colonised as part of the flora on their external genital organs and pass the bacteria on to mares during mating.

Although internal spread in the stallion is rare, the bacteria may occasionally invade the urethra and sex glands, causing pus and bacteria to contaminate the semen.

4. How is infection prevented and controlled?

The main ways of preventing infection are:

- check stallions and mares for infection before they are mated: this is done through swabbing
- if a horse proves to be infected, do not use it for mating until the infection has been successfully treated
- always exercise strict hygiene measures when handling mares and stallions.

The main ways of stopping the spread of infection if it does occur are to:

- stop mating by the infected horse(s)
- treat the infection and re-swab to check that the infection has cleared up before resuming mating
- exercise strict hygiene measures when handling the horses involved.

5. CEM is a notifiable disease

In the UK, isolation of the CEM organism is notifiable by law, meaning that a suspicion or isolation of the organism must be reported to a Divisional Veterinary Officer (DVO) of the Ministry of Agriculture, Fisheries and Food (MAFF).

This is a statutory requirement under the Infectious Diseases of Horses Order 1987. Copies of the Order (reference: 1987 No. 790) are obtainable from HMSO.

6. Hygiene

Owing to the risk of indirect infection, stud staff should be made aware that

CEM, *Klebsiella pneumoniae* and *Pseudomonas aeruginosa* can be highly contagious. Staff should wear disposable gloves at all times when handling the genitalia of mares and stallions, and should change gloves between each horse.

Separate utensils should be used for each stallion.

If mares are infected when pregnant or foaling, hygiene is very important to prevent the transmission of infection through contaminated utensils or discharges from the mare.

7. Swabbing

Swabbing requirements are different for the stallion and mare. For the mare they vary, depending on whether she has been previously infected or exposed to risk of infection. Where this is the case, mares are classified 'high risk'. Otherwise, they are classified 'low risk' – see Section 8.

For **mares** there are two types of swab:

'Endometrial swab': a swab taken during early oestrus from the lining of the uterus via the cervix

'Clitoral swab': a swab taken from the clitoral fossa, including the clitoral sinuses.

For **stallions** 'a set of swabs' includes samples from the urethra, urethral fossa and penile sheath, plus pre-ejaculatory fluid when possible.

Swabs from both mares and stallions should be taken each year after 1st January. The swabs should be sent immediately to an Approved Laboratory (see pages 213–14) which will return the results on an official Laboratory Certificate (see page 215). The Laboratory should culture all swabs aerobically and microaerophilically to screen for CEMO, *Klebsiella pneumoniae* (capsule types 1, 2 and 5) and *Pseudomonas aeruginosa.*

8. 'Low risk' and 'High risk' mares

'High risk' ares are:

(a) mares from which CEMO has been isolated since 1989
(b) mares from which CEMO was isolated before 1989 and which have not since been mated
(c) mares mated with any stallions which transmitted CEM in 1995
(d) mares arriving from countries other than Canada, France, Germany, Ireland, Italy, the UK and the USA, if mated with stallions resident outside these countries in 1995
(e) barren and maiden mares arriving from countries other than Canada, France, Germany, Ireland, Italy, the UK and the USA.

NB: Information on the identity of high risk Thoroughbred mares can be obtained from the organisations listed on pages 214 and 216.

Low-risk mares are any mares not defined as high risk.

NB: Mares which have been mated in Canada, France, Germany, Ireland, Italy, the UK or the USA, which have then gone to other countries and which subsequently return to one of these countries are 'low risk' providing they have not been mated again in a high risk country. However, additional swabbing may be carried out as an extra precaution.

9. Preventing infection – recommendations for 1996

A. *Stallions*

After 1st January and before the start of the breeding season, stallion studs should, for all stallions and teasers:

- Take two sets of swabs, at intervals of no less than 7 days.
- Complete a Stallion Certificate (example on page 218).

NB: Do not mate until ALL the swab results are available.

First season stallions warrant additional precautions. The first mares mated with them should be screened thoroughly for bacterial reproductive infections by post-mating clitoral and endometrial swabbing under veterinary direction.

Stallion studs should receive, for each mare booked in, a Mare Certificate and, where appropriate, Laboratory Certificate(s) before the mare arrives. Advance Laboratory Certificate requirements are detailed in Section B below.

B. *Mares*

Before mares are moved to the stallion stud farm, owners should classify them as 'high risk' or 'low risk', then:

- complete a Mare Certificate (example on page 219)
- carry out any swabbing to be done at the home premises and await the Laboratory Certificate
- send the Mare Certificate and any Laboratory Certificate to the stallion stud farm. Ensure that certification is received there before the mare arrives.

Swabbing requirements are as follows:

'Low risk' mares – resident at stallion stud

Before first mating:

- Clitoral swab on arrival at stallion stud[1]
- Endometrial swab during oestrus at stallion stud.

Mating in subsequent oestrous periods:

- Repeat endometrial swab as above.

[1] This swab may be taken at the home premises by agreement with the

stallion stud. The Laboratory Certificate must be sent to the stallion stud before the mare arrives.

'High risk' mares – resident at stallion stud
Before first mating:

- Clitoral swab before arrival at stallion stud[2]
- Clitoral swab on arrival at stallion stud
- Endometrial swab during oestrus at stallion stud.

Mating in subsequent oestrous periods:

- Repeat endometrial swab as above.

[2] The Laboratory Certificate must be sent to the stallion stud before the mare arrives.
NB: Do not mate until ALL the swab results are available.

'Low risk' mares – walking in
Before the mare is first walked in:

- Clitoral swab[3]
- Endometrial swab during oestrus.[3]

Walkings in during subsequent oestrous periods:

- Repeat endometrial swab as above.

[3] The Laboratory Certificates must be sent to the stallion stud before the mare is walked in.

'High risk' mares – walking in
Before the mare is first walked in:

- Clitoral swab before arrival at boarding stud[4]
- Clitoral swab on arrival at boarding stud[4]
- Endometrial swab during oestrus at boarding stud.[4]

Walkings in during subsequent oestrous periods:

- Repeat endometrial swab as above.

[4] Laboratory Certificate from first clitoral swab – send to the boarding stud before the mare arrives.
Laboratory Certificates from all swabs – send to the stallion stud before the mare is walked in.
NB: Do not mate until ALL the swab results are available.

Important notes on swabs

Results of swabs: for 'low risk' mares, the stallion stud manager may, on veterinary advice, allow mating to proceed on the basis of satisfactory results from aerobic culture of endometrial swabs if adequate clitoral swabbing has already been carried out. The microaerophilic endometrial swab results should still be sent to the stallion stud as soon as they are available. For 'high risk' mares, ALL results must be confirmed as negative before mating commences.

Clitoral swabs: in the case of pregnant mares, these swabs may be taken before or after foaling.

Endometrial swabs: a negative result remains valid during the oestrous period in which the mare is mated and subsequently if she is not mated. If she does not conceive on first mating, a repeat swab should be taken during all subsequent oestrous periods prior to further mating.

Abnormal return to service (all mares)

If mares come back into season at unusual times, a full set of swabs must be taken and cultured under aerobic and microaerophilic conditions.

Boarding of 'high risk' mares

High risk walking in mares should be boarded at a farm which is under control by or meets full approval of the stallion stud. The veterinary practices involved should liaise closely to ensure adherence to the Code of Practice and to arrange any additional precautions.

If CEM is confirmed on a boarding farm where a 'high risk' mare resides or at a stallion stud she has visited, no mares should be moved from the boarding farm until all have been swabbed with negative results.

Foaling of 'high risk' mares

Mares infected with CEM must be foaled in isolation. The placenta must be disposed of hygienically.

Foals born to known infected mares should be swabbed three times, at intervals of not less than seven days, before three months of age:

- Filly foals: swab the clitoral fossa
- Colt foals: swab inside the penile sheath and around the tip of the penis.

10. Controlling infection – recommendations for 1996

When infection is suspected or confirmed, mating must cease until treatment has taken place under veterinary direction and subsequent swabbing has proved that the infection has cleared up. The first swabs should be taken seven or more days after the treatment has ended. Repeat clitoral and penile swabs should subsequently be taken at intervals of seven or more days. Repeat endometrial swabs should ideally be collected during the next three oestrous periods.

In countries where CEM is notifiable, the government must be informed (for the UK, see Section 5 above). You should also inform your breeders' association.

If the CEM organism is suspected or confirmed in mares or stallions prior to mating:

(a) Seek veterinary advice and notify the DVO of MAFF IMMEDIATELY.
(b) Isolate the mares or stallions and treat as advised by the Veterinary Surgeon.

If the CEM organism is suspected or confirmed in mares or stallions after mating:

(a) Seek veterinary advice and notify the DVO of MAFF IMMEDIATELY.
(b) Stop mating by the stallion.
(c) Isolate and treat the stallion under veterinary direction.
(d) Isolate and treat the infected mares as advised by the Veterinary Surgeon.
(e) Check and deal with any other mares implicated in the outbreak as advised by the Veterinary Surgeon; this may include blood tests.
(f) Notify all owners of mares booked to the stallion, including any which have already left the stud.
(g) Notify the breeders' association.
(h) Do not resume mating by the stallion until negative results from three full post-treatment sets of swabs have been obtained; the stallion should also be test mated to at least three mares.

11. Export certification (UK)

Swabs taken for examination for CEMO from horses in the UK prior to export must be sent to one of the export approved laboratories of the Ministry of Agriculture, Fisheries and Food. These are the Central Veterinary Laboratories in Weybridge and Lasswade, and the Veterinary Investigation Centre in Bury St Edmunds.

12. *Klebsiella pneumoniae* and *Pseudomonas aeruginosa*

The means of spread of infection and the signs and stages of infection with *Klebsiella pneumoniae* and *Pseudomonas aeruginosa* are similar to those described for CEMO in Sections 2 and 3 above, but infection may also become established in the bladder and urinary system.

Infection by these bacteria can be prevented by implementing the same measures as for CEM (Sections 4, 6, 7 and 9 above). All swabs should therefore be screened for these bacteria as well as for CEMO.

If infection is confirmed in mares:

- Isolate and treat mares under veterinary advice.

If infection is confirmed in stallions:

- Stop mating
- Isolate, treat and swab under veterinary direction.

The Veterinary Surgeon should advise on the resumption of mating in both cases.

There are many different capsule types of *K. pneumoniae*, most of which are not considered to be pathogenic in the true venereal sense. However, types 1, 2 and 5 (venereal types) are considered to be pathogenic and may be sexually transmitted. Therefore, when *K. pneumoniae* is identified from mares and stallions, the tests necessary to determine which capsule type(s) is (are) present must be undertaken and then advice from a specialist laboratory and/or Veterinary Surgeon must be sought.

There are a number of strains of *P. aeruginosa*, not all of which cause true venereal disease and there is, as yet, no reliable laboratory test to differentiate between the strains. All isolates must therefore be considered as potential venereal pathogens unless proved otherwise by test mating. When transmitted to the stallion's penis, *P. aeruginosa* can be extremely difficult to eradicate.

APPROVED LABORATORIES

Information on laboratories approved for testing for CEM is available from the following organisations.

France

Ministère de l'Agriculture et de la Forêt,
Direction Générale de l'Alimentation,
175 rue du Chevaleret,
75646 Paris cedex 13
Telephone: (1) 49 55 84 55; telefax: (1) 45 86 63 08.

Germany

Direktorium für Vollblutzucht und Rennen eV,
Rennbahnstrasse 154,
50737 Koln 60
Telephone: (221) 749 8113; telefax: (221) 749 8104.

Ireland

Department of Agriculture and Food,
Abbotstown,
Castleknock,
Dublin 15
Telephone: (1) 607 2000; telefax: (1) 821 3010.

Italy

Istituto Malattie Infettive,
Facolta di Medicina Veterinaria,
V Celoria 10
Milano
Telephone: (2) 23 66 474.

United Kingdom

Horserace Betting Levy Board,
52 Grosvenor Gardens,
London SW1W 0AU
Telephone: 0171 333 0043; telefax: 0171 333 0041.

A list of laboratories approved in the UK by the Horserace Betting Levy Board is published annually in December, in the *Veterinary Record*.

HIGH RISK MARES

Information on the identity of high risk mares should be obtainable from the following organisations.

France

Syndicat des Eleveurs de Chevaux de Sang de France,
257 rue du Jour se Lève,
92100 Boulogne
Telephone: (1) 47 61 06 09; telefax: (1) 47 61 06 74.

Ministère de l'Agriculture et de la Forêt,
Direction Générale de l'Alimentation,
175 rue du Chevaleret,
75646 Paris cedex 13
Telephone: (1) 49 55 84 55; telefax: (1) 45 86 63 08.

Germany

Direktorium für Vollblutzucht und Rennen eV
Rennbahnstrasse 154
50737 Koln 60
Telephone: (221) 749 8113; telefax: (221) 749 8104.

Ireland

The Irish Thoroughbred Breeders' Association,
Old Connell House,
Newbridge,
Co. Kildare
Telephone: (45) 31890.

LABORATORY CERTIFICATE (FOR USE IN THE UK DURING THE 1996 SEASON)

For use only by Approved Laboratories* December 1995 – November 1996.

Swabs contained in transport medium and labelled as collected from the stallion/mare:

....

from the following sites: ....

....

were submitted by ....

for bacteriological examination on (date[s]) ....

I ....

of (Laboratory) ....

certify that the above swabs were examined under specific conditions of microaerophilic and aerobic culture with the following results:

Taylorella equigenitalis (CEMO) **WAS/WAS NOT**** isolated
Pseudomonas aeruginosa **WAS/WAS NOT**** isolated
Klebsiella pneumoniae **WAS†/WAS NOT**** isolated
Where *K. pneumoniae* was isolated, capsule type(s) identified were

....

NAME AND QUALIFICATIONS (PLEASE PRINT) ....

SIGNATURE .... DATE ....

LABORATORY NAME AND ADDRESS ....

....

....

....

* An Approved Laboratory is one whose name is published in the Veterinary Record by the Horserace Betting Levy Board in December 1995.
** Delete as appropriate.
† In the event of a positive *Klebsiella pneumoniae* isolate, capsule typing should be performed and the results detailed to aid the determination of potential venereal pathogenicity.

Italy

Associazione Nazionale Allevatori Cavalli Purosangue,
Via del Caravaggio 3,
20144 Milano
Telephone: (2) 48 01 20 02 or 49 80 589; telefax: (2) 48 19 45 47.

United Kingdom

Thoroughbred Breeders' Association,
Stanstead House,
The Avenue,
Newmarket,
Suffolk
Telephone: 01638 661321; telefax: 01638 665621.

COMMON CODE OF PRACTICE FOR EQUINE VIRAL ARTERITIS

1. What is EVA?

Equine viral arteritis (EVA) is a contagious disease caused by the equine arteritis virus (EAV). The virus occurs worldwide and is present in Great Britain and every mainland European country.

The virus may cause abortion or pregnancy failure in mares.

EVA may be fatal.

2. How does the infection spread?

A. Routes of infection

Infection spreads through transmission of the virus between horses in two main ways:

- venereal infection of mares by stallions during mating
- by direct contact in droplets (e.g. from coughing and snorting) from the respiratory tract.

B. The shedder stallion

The stallion is a very important source of the virus. On infection, the virus localises in his accessory sex glands and he will shed the virus in his semen for several weeks afterwards, or for many months or years and possibly for life. After recovery from acute illness, his fertility is not affected and he will show no further clinical signs of infection even though he may still be infectious. Shedder stallions will infect susceptible mares during mating and these mares may, in turn, infect in-contact animals via the respiratory route.

It is important to note that the shedder stallion is always seropositive (i.e. past or existing infection indicated in a blood test) but that a seropositive stallion is not necessarily a shedder.

Breeders using AI must note that the virus can survive in chilled and frozen semen.

C. Mares

Present available evidence indicates that the 'carrier' state does not occur in mares.

3. What are the symptoms of EVA?

The variety and severity of clinical signs of EVA vary widely. Infection may be obvious or there may be no signs at all. Even when there are no signs, infection can still be transmitted and stallions might still become shedders.

The main signs that are seen include fever, lethargy, depression, swelling of the lower legs, conjunctivitis ('pink eye'), swelling around the eye socket and upper eyelid, nasal discharge, 'nettle rash' and swelling of the scrotum and mammary gland. In pregnant mares, abortion may occur.

4. How is the disease diagnosed?

Because of the variability or the possible absence of symptoms, clinical diagnosis is not always possible.

Laboratory diagnosis is therefore essential. This requires appropriate samples, which are nasopharyngeal swabs, heparinised blood, semen, serum and possibly urine, to be taken by a Veterinary Surgeon and sent to a specialist laboratory.

In blood samples, laboratories look for antibodies to the virus (serological test); in other samples, they look for the virus itself (virus isolation test).

Where abortion may be EVA-related, detailed clinical information must be sent to the laboratory with the fetus and its membranes.

5. How is EVA treated?

There is no treatment available for EVA itself, although there may be treatments to alleviate some of its symptoms.

6. How can EVA be avoided?

The main ways of preventing infection are:

- test horses imported from abroad
- test horses in this country at the beginning of the breeding season
- if a horse proves to be infected, do not use it for mating until it is no longer infectious.

For Britain and Ireland, there is one vaccine licensed for use in all horses, but see page 224 for more information. Vaccination causes horses to become seropositive. Therefore, horses **must** be blood tested before being vaccinated to show that they were seronegative before the vaccine was given. No vaccines are licensed in any other member state of the European Union (EU) but there is a vaccine available in a limited number of non-EU countries.

CONTAGIOUS EQUINE METRITIS AND OTHER EQUINE BACTERIAL VENEREAL DISEASES (1996 SEASON)

Stallion certificate

Certificate of examination of stallions to be completed by a Veterinary Surgeon.

On the following two dates (1) ....

(2) ....

swabs were obtained from the penile sheath, the urethra, the urethral fossa and a sample of the pre-ejaculatory fluid from the stallion named ....

passport number (where available) ....

and submitted for bacteriological examination for *Taylorella equigenitalis* (CEMO), *Klebsiella pneumoniae* and *Pseudomonas aeruginosa* at the ....

Approved Laboratory and gave negative results.

SIGNATURE ....

MRCVS

NAME (PLEASE PRINT) ....

ADDRESS ....

....

....

....

DATE ....

CONTAGIOUS EQUINE METRITIS AND OTHER EQUINE BACTERIAL VENEREAL DISEASES (1996 SEASON)

Mare certificate

Certificate to be completed by mare owner and lodged with the prospective stallion stud farm owner before the mare is sent to the stallion stud farm.

Name of mare ....

Passport number (where available) ....

Name and address of owner ....

....

....

1993 stud visited ....

mated with .... result ....

1994 stud visited ....

mated with .... result ....

1995 stud visited ....

mated with .... result ....

Additional information including the results of positive bacteriological examinations for *CEMO, Klebsiella pneumoniae* and *Pseudomonas aeruginosa* at any time:

....

....

NAME (PLEASE PRINT) ....

SIGNATURE ....

DATE ....

7. EVA is a notifiable disease

In Great Britain, EVA is a notifiable disease in certain circumstances under the Equine Viral Arteritis Order 1995.

The notification requirements are complex but, essentially, it is a legal requirement to notify a Divisional Veterinary Officer (DVO) of the Ministry of Agriculture, Fisheries and Food (MAFF) when:

- it is known or suspected that a stallion has the disease or is a carrier of the virus
- it is known or suspected that a mare which has been mated or subjected to Artificial Insemination in the last 14 days has become infected with the virus.

Full details of the exact notification requirements are in the Order, which is obtainable from HMSO (reference: 1995 No. 1755).

8. Preventing infection – recommendations for 1996

A. Imported horses

Where it is intended to import horses, semen or embryos, veterinary or other specialist advice should be taken on the incidence of EVA in the exporting country. As a general guide, the importer should take the following precautions if the horse is imported from a country where EVA is known or suspected to occur.

- As a condition of the purchase agreement, require that the horse is tested for EVA before leaving the country of origin. The samples should be sent to a competent laboratory, which does not need to be in the country of origin.
- Place the horse in isolation immediately on arrival and keep it there for at least 21 days. Blood samples should be taken on arrival and at least 14 days later and sent to a competent laboratory for examination for antibodies to EAV. When the results are available, consult your Veterinary Surgeon about the next steps.
- When importing semen for use in AI, establish the status of the donor stallion at the time when the semen was collected. If the stallion was seropositive, the semen should not be used unless it can be proved that he was not a shedder.
- When importing embryos, establish the status of both the stallion and mare at the time of conception. For mares, seronegative status, or seropositive status with stable or declining EAV antibody levels, is required. For stallions, seronegative status, or seropositive status with proof that they are not shedders, is required.

B. Stallions

After 1st January in any year, all **UNVACCINATED STALLIONS AND**

TEASERS should be serologically tested. Do not use them for mating until the results are available.

If the stallion is seronegative, mating may begin.

If the stallion is seropositive, he may be a shedder and must be isolated while steps are taken to determine whether or not he is shedding virus in his semen – see page 223 for testing methods. He must not be used for mating or AI during this time.

If he proves to be a shedder, he must remain in isolation until shedding stops or his future is decided.

VACCINATED STALLIONS AND TEASERS may be seropositive or seronegative, depending on when the last course of vaccine was given and on whether the horse might have become infected since the effect of the vaccine wore off. These horses should be blood tested after 1st January. Do not use them for mating until the results are available.

If the stallion is seronegative, mating may begin.

If he is seropositive, his history in the past 12 months – including dates of EVA vaccinations, results of pre-vaccination blood testing and contacts with other horses since the last vaccination – should be reviewed. If there is any possibility that his seropositive status is the result of infection rather than vaccination, he should be isolated and further tested to determine whether he is shedding virus in his semen – see page 223 for test methods. He must not be used for mating or AI at this time.

C. Mares

The risk associated with any mare can vary. Decisions regarding the testing of mares visiting stallions should therefore be made at local level, in consultation with the Veterinary Surgeon, according to the circumstances of individual studfarms and the mare's history and contacts with other horses in the past year.

In any breeding season, the safest way to avoid risk is to blood test all mares within 4 weeks before mating. Foster mares should also be tested. Do not mate the mare until the results are available.

If a mare is seronegative, mating may begin. If she is seropositive, she must be isolated – preferably off the stallion stud – until her EAV antibody levels are stable or declining. In-contacts should be isolated and screened for EAV.

D. Foaling – seropositive mares

Any pregnant seropositive mares should be foaled in isolation unless the vaccination or infection which caused seropositivity occurred before the pregnancy. If in any doubt, consult the Veterinary Surgeon.

E. Abortion and newborn foal death

If there is any possibility that EVA caused an abortion or newborn foal death, the fetus or carcase together with appropriate samples from the mare's placenta and her clinical history must be sent immediately to a competent laboratory for specific examination.

F. Artificial insemination

The equine arteritis virus survives in chilled and frozen semen and is *not* affected by the antibiotics added to semen. Donor stallions must therefore be checked according to Section B above.

The stallion stud must record the dates of collection of semen and its movement to other premises.

G. Sport horses

It is thought that there is a particular risk of EVA transmission associated with the international movement of sport horse stallions. Precautions are therefore needed when these are used for mating or semen collection for AI. Where these stallions are imported from any member state of the European Union (EU), they are not required to undergo any official EVA testing. Their EVA status must therefore be established privately before mating or semen collection. The British Government lays down official EVA testing requirements for all stallions imported from non-EU countries. However, additional private testing may be carried out as a further precaution.

If a stallion is normally resident in this country, testing should be repeated each time he returns from international competition.

Mares and stallions in this category may readily acquire EVA through the respiratory route.

9. Controlling infection – recommendations for 1996

If EVA occurs:

(a) Seek veterinary advice and notify the DVO of MAFF IMMEDIATELY.
(b) Stop movement on/off the premises.
(c) Stop mating.
(d) Stop semen collection for AI; check stored semen (one dose of each batch to be tested by a competent laboratory).
(e) Isolate clinical cases and their in-contacts. Take samples for virus isolation tests by a competent laboratory.
(f) Screen all horses at the premises by blood testing. Healthy seronegative animals which have been in contact with the clinical cases should be grouped away from other healthy seronegative horses.
(g) Notify:

- owners of horses at and due to arrive at the premises
- owners of horses which have left the premises
- recipients of semen from the premises
- your breeders' association.

(h) Repeat blood testing after 14 days and again every 14 days until the outbreak is over. If any previously healthy or seronegative horses become ill or become seropositive, move them into the appropriate group.
(i) Keep seropositive horses in isolation for at least one month.
(j) If stallions remain seropositive, steps must be taken to determine whether they are shedders. See below. Stallions which prove to be shedders must be kept in strict isolation until their future is decided and must not be used for mating or semen collection during this time.
(k) Clean and disinfect stables and vehicles used for horse transport.
(l) Good hygiene must be exercised. If possible, separate staff should be used for the different groups of horses.
(m) Take veterinary advice on the resumption of movement and breeding activity.
(n) Pregnant mares must be isolated for at least one month after leaving the premises. Those remaining on the premises should be kept in isolation for at least one month after active infection has stopped.

Identifying shedder stallions

When a seropositive stallion is identified, it is vital to establish whether he is shedding EAV in his semen. If so, he is a primary source of infection.

The stallion must be kept in strict isolation for at least a month. The following methods should be used to determine whether he is a shedder:

1. Virus isolation

Collect two whole ejaculates of semen at intervals of at least seven days and send them to a competent laboratory. Transport requirements (e.g. cooling) should be arranged with the laboratory.

2. Test mating

This must be done only in strict isolation. The stallion and mares must be kept away from *all* contact with other horses. Apply the following procedure:

- Identify at least two seronegative mares.
- Take and store blood samples from each; then isolate the mares.
- Mate each mare twice a day with the stallion on two consecutive days.
- Keep the mares in isolation.
- After 28 days, take blood samples and send them, with the pre-isolation samples, to a competent laboratory for a virus isolation test.

If the mares remain seronegative, the stallion is unlikely to be a shedder and can be released after a clinical examination.

If one or more mares becomes seropositive, the stallion is a shedder and must be kept in isolation. He must not be used for mating or AI as long as he is still shedding.

Seropositive mares must remain in isolation until they are no longer infectious.

3. Review of recent history of mares

Subject unvaccinated mares which have recently been mated to the stallion to veterinary clinical examination and blood testing. If they show clinical signs of EVA or have become seropositive after mating, the stallion may be a shedder.

This method is insufficient on its own to confirm shedding and should be used with one or both of the other methods.

Stallions which are shedders must be kept in isolation until their future is decided.

Options include:

euthanasia
castration (followed by 6 weeks' isolation).

NB: FOR GREAT BRITAIN, THE OPTIONS ARE LAID DOWN BY THE EVA ORDER 1995.

EVA vaccine

A vaccine (Artervac, Willows Francis) is available on an Animal Test Certificate for all horses in the UK.

There are data to show that Artervac is safe. There is also experimental efficacy data to show that it can protect horses three weeks after the second dose of vaccine is given. However, it is not yet clear how the vaccine will perform in the field. If it performs well, it will be an effective way of protecting stallions.

Vaccinated horses will become seropositive. Horses should therefore be blood tested before vaccination to show that they were previously seronegative. The following records, certified by a Veterinary Surgeon, should be kept:

- date when pre-vaccination blood sample was taken
- certificate from laboratory showing blood test result
- date when vaccination was given and batch number of the vaccine.

These records are important as evidence of previous seronegativity for breeding *and* export purposes. Some importing countries require this information for vaccinated horses, either in passports or official export certificates.

As the vaccine's efficacy is not yet fully known, owners should monitor the horse's antibody response after vaccination, in consultation with the Veterinary Surgeon.

VACCINATION IS NOT AN ALTERNATIVE TO GOOD MANAGEMENT

THE CODE OF PRACTICE REMAINS ESSENTIAL TO PREVENT EVA

CODE OF PRACTICE FOR EQUID HERPESVIRUS-1

1. What is EHV-1?

EHV-1 is a common and contagious virus which causes abortion, respiratory disease and paralysis.

It should be noted that EHV-4 can also cause abortion but more usually causes respiratory disease only.

2. How does infection occur?

All classes of horses and ponies can be a source of EHV-1. Pregnant mares should therefore be kept separate from all other stock to avoid infection which may lead to abortion and to disease in live foals.

The virus usually spreads via the respiratory tract, but aborted fetuses, fetal membranes and fluids are a particularly dangerous source of infection. All aborted fetuses and carcases from newborn foal deaths must therefore be handled hygienically and sent to a competent laboratory for examination.

Infected foals can pass on infection, via the respiratory route, to healthy mares, other foals and other in-contacts.

Mares which have aborted or whose foal has died are a source of infection to other foals and horses, also via the respiratory route.

Healthy foals can become infected from any horses as well as infected mares and foals.

Mares and other horses can be 'carriers' of the virus, meaning that they may transmit infection without showing signs of illness themselves. Illness may become apparent in carriers from time to time, especially after stress or after suffering another disease. The virus is always contagious at this time.

The virus can survive in the environment for several weeks; indirect infection is therefore possible.

3. When does abortion occur?

Abortion usually occurs in late pregnancy (8–11 months) but can be as early as four months.

Following infection, abortion can happen from two weeks to several months later.

Prolonged transport and other types of stress during late pregnancy may increase the risk of infection of the fetus.

4. What about live infected foals?

Infected foals are usually abnormal from birth, showing weakness, jaundice, difficulty in breathing and occasionally nervous symptoms. They usually die within three days.

These foals are highly contagious through direct contact via the respiratory route and through shedding virus into the environment. All horses can become infected but mares which have recently foaled are probably at greatest risk.

5. What about respiratory disease?

EHV-1 usually causes respiratory disease in weaned foals and yearlings, most often in autumn and winter. However, older animals can succumb. These are more likely than the younger animals to transmit the virus without showing signs of infection.

The signs that are seen are mild fever, coughing, discharge from the nose and other signs of respiratory disease.

6. How is EHV-1 diagnosed?

The presence of EHV-1 can only be diagnosed in a laboratory.

For abortion and newborn foal death, the laboratory requires the fetus or foal carcase. Blood testing the mare is *not* appropriate for diagnosing an EHV-1 abortion.

Members of the Thoroughbred Breeders' Association in Great Britain are reminded that a contribution may be available towards laboratory costs for aborted fetuses or foals which die within 14 days of birth. Further details are available from the TBA.

For confirmation of EHV-1 as the cause of respiratory disease or paralysis, blood samples and swabs from the throat are required.

7. Is EHV-1 notifiable?

There are no legal notification requirements for EHV-1 in the UK.

However, because the disease is spread easily between horses and can have severe consequences, it is **very important** to alert owners of horses which might be at risk of infection or might spread infection away from your premises following an outbreak at your premises. These owners can then arrange to take their own precautions against the spread of infection at their premises. Recommendations for reporting are given in Section 9 below.

On no account should any horse known or suspected to have disease caused by EHV-1 be sent, during the breeding season, to a stallion stud or to other premises where there are pregnant mares or brood mares.

8. Preventing EHV-1 – recommendations for 1996

A. Management

Where possible, mares should foal at home and go to the stallion with a healthy foal at foot.

Where this is not possible, pregnant mares should arrive at the stallion stud ideally one month before foaling is due. They should be put in isolated groups with other healthy pregnant mares; these groups should be as small as possible. Mares in late pregnancy and those from sales yards and abroad are a particular risk and should be isolated alone.

The isolated groups and individuals should be separated as far as possible from weaned foals, yearlings, horses out of training and competition horses. Fillies out of training are a particular risk to pregnant mares.

Mares in late pregnancy should not travel with other stock, particularly mares which have aborted recently.

If a foster mare is brought to the stud, she should be isolated – particularly from pregnant mares – until it has been proved that her own foal's death was not caused by EHV-1.

Stallions should ideally be housed in premises separate to the mare operations.

B. Hygiene

EHV-1 is destroyed readily by heat and disinfectants. Stables and vehicles for horse transport should therefore be cleaned and disinfected regularly as a matter of routine, using approved disinfectants and steam cleaning. If cleaning and disinfection are inadequate, the virus may survive in the environment for several weeks.

Ideally, separate staff should deal with separate groups of mares. If this is not possible, pregnant mares should be handled first each day.

C. Vaccination

One vaccine (Pneumabort-K, Willows Francis) is licensed for use against abortion in the UK. This appears to be a useful aid in preventing multiple abortion. Vaccination of mares should therefore be considered.

Another vaccine (Duvaxyn, Solvay Duphar) is licensed for use against the respiratory form of EHV-1 and EHV-4 in the UK.

Vaccination of all horses/ponies on any stud using these vaccines under veterinary direction may be advantageous to raise the level of protection against EHV-1. However, this may not necessarily provide total protection.

VACCINATION IS NOT AN ALTERNATIVE TO GOOD MANAGEMENT

THE CODE OF PRACTICE REMAINS ESSENTIAL TO PREVENT EHV-1

9. Controlling EHV-1 – recommendations for 1996

A. *If: – abortion occurs*
– a foal is born dead
– a foal is born ill
– a foal becomes ill within 14 days of birth:

(a) Seek veterinary advice IMMEDIATELY.
(b) For abortions and foals born dead:

- place the mare in strict isolation
- send the fetus and its membranes or the foal carcase to a competent laboratory for examination as instructed by the Veterinary Surgeon; use leakproof containers.

(c) For sick live foals:

- place the mare and foal in strict isolation
- send samples (usually nasopharyngeal swabs and heparinised blood) to a competent laboratory for examination as instructed by the Veterinary Surgeon; use leakproof containers
- the attendant should have no contact with pregnant mares.

(d) Stop movement off the stud. Do not allow any pregnant mare onto the stud until EHV-1 has been excluded as the cause of the abortion or foal death or illness.
(e) Notify owners due to send mares to the stud.
(f) Disinfect and destroy bedding; clean and disinfect premises and vehicles used for horse transport under veterinary supervision.
(g) If preliminary laboratory results indicate EHV-1, divide pregnant mares in the contact group into even smaller groups to minimise the spread of any infection (**NB:** some may still abort).

B. *If EHV-1 is confirmed:*

(a) Maintain isolation and movement restrictions and hygiene measures.
(b) Notify:

- Your breeders' association
  by telephone
  in writing.
- Owners (or their agents) of:
  mares at the stud
  mares due to be sent to the stud.
- Others:
  premises to which mares from the stud have been sent
  premises to which mares from the stud are to be sent.

Notification is extremely important. Failure to notify the disease can contribute to the spread of infection to the detriment of all owners and their horses, particularly mare owners.

C. *After EHV-1 abortion at a stallion stud:*

(a) The stud can accept barren mares, maiden mares and mares which have produced healthy foals at home, providing there is no sign of infection at the home premises.
(b) Non-pregnant mares which have been on the stud can visit other premises after one month from the date of the last abortion, providing they can be isolated from all pregnant mares for at least two months at the premises they are visiting.*
(c) Pregnant mares due to foal in the current season must stay at the stud until they foal.
(d) Walking-in mares can visit the stud, but cannot return to their boarding studs until one month after the last clinical case has occurred.*
(e) Mares which have aborted must be kept in isolation from mares in late pregnancy for eight weeks after abortion. Present evidence indicates low risk of spread of infection if mares are mated on the second heat cycle after abortion.
(f) Mares that returned home pregnant from such studs where abortion occurred the previous season should foal in isolation at home. Where this is not possible, the stud to which the mare is to be sent in the current season must be informed so that precautions can be taken.

* The managers and Veterinary Surgeons of the stallion stud and other premises must agree these arrangements before the mares are moved.

D. *If paralytic EHV-1 is suspected in any horse:*

(a) Seek veterinary advice IMMEDIATELY.
(b) Stop mating.
(c) Stop all movement on and off the stud.
(d) Send samples as directed by the Veterinary Surgeon to a competent laboratory for examination; use leakproof containers.
(e) Divide horses into small groups, keeping pregnant mares separate from all others.
(f) Implement A(e), A(f) and B above.

E. *If paralytic EHV-1 is confirmed*

Policy should be decided with the Veterinary Surgeon. This should include screening and clearance of each group before individuals in the group return home. Individuals should then be isolated at home, especially pregnant mares, until after foaling.

ISOLATION

The Codes of Practice often refer to the isolation of horses. These notes offer guidance on isolation.

In its most rigorous sense, 'strict isolation' means a separate facility with separate staff, separate protective clothing, separate utensils/equipment, and thorough steam cleaning and disinfection of stables between each occupant. A rigorous interpretation, published by the Tripartite Group of the veterinary services of the Governments of France, Great Britain and Ireland, is as follows:

Premises

1. Isolation on a stud or breeding premises is not recommended.
2. The isolation premises must be a separate, enclosed building of sound, permanent construction, capable of being effectively cleansed and disinfected.
3. It must not be possible for other horses to approach within 100 metres of the isolation premises while they are in use.
4. An adequate supply of water must be available at all times for the isolated horses and for cleaning purposes.
5. Adequate supplies of food and bedding material for the whole of the isolation period must be made available and stored within the isolation premises before isolation commences.
6. Equipment and utensils used for feeding, grooming and cleansing must be used only in the isolation premises during the isolation period.
7. Protective clothing to be used exclusively in the isolation premises must be available at the entrance to the isolation premises.

Procedures

1. Before use, all fixed and moveable equipment and utensils for feeding, grooming and cleaning within the isolation premises must be disinfected using an approved disinfectant.
2. Attendants of the isolated horses must have no contact with any other horses during the isolation period and the isolated horses have no contact, direct or indirect, with other horses.
3. The isolation period for all isolated horses shall be deemed to start from the time of entry of the last horse.
4. No person may enter the isolation premises unless specifically authorised to do so.
5. When no attendants are on duty, the premises must be locked securely to prevent the entry of unauthorised persons.

If such strict measures are not possible in practice, studs should devise their own isolation programme and procedures in consultation with the Veterinary Surgeon. These should include, for example:

- The designation of a yard and associated paddock as an isolation area in a geographically separate area of the stud.
- The designation of individual staff to work in the isolation facility with separate protective clothing and recognised disinfectants as and when

required. These individuals should either not be involved with work on the rest of the stud farm during periods of isolation, or they should work in the isolation area only after they have finished the rest of the stud.
- The establishment, for use when required, of 'standard procedures', the precise details of which might be varied with the disease condition in question, following consultation between the stud manager and the attending Veterinary Surgeon.

TRANSPORT

There is potential for transmission of infectious diseases during transport.

Cleanliness and hygiene on board all forms of transport are the responsibility of the vehicle owner in private transport and the vehicle operator in contracted transport. The following notes are for guidance in either case.

- Vehicles should be cleaned and disinfected frequently and regularly, preferably using recognised viricidal disinfectants.
- Vehicles should be clean before horses are loaded.
- Prior vaccination of horses may reduce the risk of disease transmission during transport.
- When mixed loads are unavoidable, give careful consideration to the categories of horses which are transported together so as to minimise the risk (e.g. risk to pregnant mares of EHV-1 infection).
- Horses should be healthy and fit to travel.
- Sick animals should not be transported except when they are travelling, under veterinary supervision, to obtain veterinary treatment. Where transport of such horses is unavoidable, they must not be put in mixed loads without the consent of other owners (or their agents) of horses in that load. Veterinary advice may be needed.
- If horses or their in-contacts are ill on or shortly after arrival at their destination, inform the transport operator at once. The operator should inform other clients with animals in the same load. Take veterinary advice on the sick horses, isolating them if necessary.
- Facilities should, if needed, be made available for cleaning/mucking out of lorries at premises where loading/unloading stops are made.

GLOSSARY OF TERMS

This glossary explains technical terms as they are used in the Codes of Practice:

Aerobically	In the presence of oxygen
Antibody	Protective substance produced by the body in response to the presence of a virus

Antigen	Substance or organism which may be recognised by the body as being foreign to it, e.g. part of a virus or bacterium
Cervix	Neck of the uterus opening into the vagina
Clitoral	Relating to the clitoris
Clitoris	A body of tissue found just inside the vulva
Endometrial	Of the endometrium, which is tissue that forms a lining inside the uterus
Genital	Relating to reproduction (e.g. genital organs or genitalia = reproductive organs)
Heparinised blood	Blood sample which has been prevented from clotting by the addition of heparin
Jaundice	Condition in which a yellow colour can be seen in the mouth, eye and vagina
Lethargy	Dullness or drowsiness
Microaerophilically	In the virtual absence of oxygen
Nasopharyngeal swab	Swab taken from the throat, behind the nasal cavities and mouth above the soft palate
Oestrus/oestrous period	In heat or in season
Pathogenic	Capable of causing disease
Placenta	Membrane which surrounds the fetus in the uterus
Scrotum	Pouch containing the testicles
Seroconversion	Change from being seronegative to seropositive
Serological test	Testing of a blood sample by a laboratory to look for antibodies to a virus
Seronegative	No evidence of infection in a blood test
Seropositive	Past or existing infection indicated in a blood test
Serum	Clear fluid which separates from solid materials of blood after clotting
Urethra	Tube through which urine is discharged from the bladder
Uterus	Womb
Venereal disease	A sexually transmitted disease
Vulva	External opening of the vagina

Further Reading

Ginther, O.J. (1992) *Reproductive Biology of the Mare*, 2nd Edition. Equiservices, 4343 Garfoot Road, Cross Plains, Wisconsin 53528.

Ginther, O.J. (1986) *Ultrasonic Imaging and Reproductive Events in the Mare*. Equiservices, 4343 Garfoot Road, Cross Plains, Wisconsin 53528.

Jackson, P.G.G. (1995) *Handbook of Veterinary Obstetrics*. W.B. Saunders Company Ltd, London.

Males, R. & Males, V. (1977) *Foaling: Brood Mare and Foal Management*. Landsdowne Press, Sydney.

McKinnon, A.O. & Voss, J.L. (1993) *Equine Reproduction*. Lea & Febiger, Philadelphia.

Pickett, B.W., Squires, E.L. & Voss, J.L. (1981) *Normal and Abnormal Sexual Behaviour of the Equine Male*. Animal Reproduction Laboratory, Colorado State University, Fort Collins, Colorado 80523.

Rossdale, P.D. & Ricketts, S.W. (1980) *Equine Stud Farm Medicine*, 2nd Edition. Baillière Tindall, London.

Walker, D.F. & Vaughan, J.T. (1980) *Bovine and Equine Urogenital Surgery*. Lea & Febiger, Philadelphia.

Zemjanis, R. (1970) *Diagnostic and Therapeutic Techniques in Animal Reproduction*, 2nd Edition. The Williams and Wilkins Company, Baltimore.

Index